Communication Disabilities
SOURCEBOOK

SECOND EDITION

Disability Series

Communication Disabilities SOURCEBOOK

SECOND EDITION

Basic Consumer Health Information about Different Types of Communication Disorders, Their Effects on Social Interaction and Daily Life, and Recovery and Rehabilitation Strategies, including Early Intervention and Assistive Technologies

Along with Facts about Legal Rights, Protections, and Benefits for People with Communication Disabilities, Tips for Caregivers, and Resources for Additional Help and Information

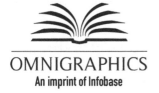

OMNIGRAPHICS
An imprint of Infobase

Bibliographic Note

Because this page cannot legibly accommodate all the copyright notices, the Bibliographic Note portion of the Preface constitutes an extension of the copyright notice.

* * *

OMNIGRAPHICS
An imprint of Infobase
8 The Green
Suite #19225
Dover, DE 19901
www.infobase.com
James Chambers, *Editorial Director*

* * *

Copyright © 2025 Infobase
ISBN 978-0-7808-2150-7
E-ISBN 978-0-7808-2151-4

Library of Congress Cataloging-in-Publication Data

Names: Chambers, James, editor.

Title: Communication disabilities sourcebook / edited by James Chambers.

Description: Second edition. | Dover, DE: Omnigraphics, an imprint of Infobase, [2024] | Series: Disability series | Includes index. | Summary: "Provides basic health information about different types of communication disorders and their effects on personal, social, and economic well-being, recovery and rehabilitation techniques, tips for caregivers, and the rights and benefits of people with communication disabilities. Includes an index and resources for additional information"-- Provided by publisher.

Identifiers: LCCN 2024031404 (print) | LCCN 2024031405 (ebook) | ISBN 9780780821507 | ISBN 9780780821514 (eISBN)

Subjects: LCSH: Communicative disorders. | People with communicative disabilities.

Classification: LCC RC423 .C635 2024 (print) | LCC RC423 (ebook) | DDC 616.85/5--dc23/eng/20240805

LC record available at https://lccn.loc.gov/2024031404

LC ebook record available at https://lccn.loc.gov/2024031405

Electronic or mechanical reproduction, including photography, recording, or any other information storage and retrieval system for the purpose of resale is strictly prohibited without permission in writing from the publisher.

The information in this publication was compiled from the sources cited and from other sources considered reliable. While every possible effort has been made to ensure reliability, the publisher will not assume liability for damages caused by inaccuracies in the data, and makes no warranty, express or implied, on the accuracy of the information contained herein.

This book is printed on acid-free paper meeting the ANSI Z39.48 Standard. The infinity symbol that appears above indicates that the paper in this book meets that standard.

Printed in the United States

Table of Contents

Preface | ix

Part 1: Understanding Communication Disorders
Chapter 1——Basics of Communication | 3
Chapter 2——The Importance of Communication and
            Its Disorders | 11
Chapter 3——Statistics on Communication Disorders | 15
Chapter 4——Disorders of Voice, Speech, and Language | 19
            Section 4.1——Voice Health and Care | 20
            Section 4.2——Hoarseness | 23
            Section 4.3——Spasmodic Dysphonia | 27
            Section 4.4——Vocal Fold Paralysis | 30
            Section 4.5——Apraxia of Speech | 32
            Section 4.6——Stuttering | 36
            Section 4.7——Developmental Language Disorder | 40
Chapter 5——Specific Language Impairment | 43
Chapter 6——Sensory Impairments Affecting Communication | 47
            Section 6.1——Hearing Disorders | 48
            Section 6.2——Low Vision | 51
Chapter 7——Central Auditory Processing Disorder | 55
Chapter 8——Other Disorders Affecting Communication | 59
            Section 8.1——Aphasia | 60
            Section 8.2——Orofacial Clefts | 62
            Section 8.3——Autism Spectrum Disorder | 65
            Section 8.4——Effects of Low Birth Weight on Communication
                         and Development | 67

Part 2: Promoting Inclusivity and Understanding
Chapter 9—Tips for Effective Interactions with People Who Have Communication Disabilities | 73
Chapter 10—The Importance of People-First Language in Discussing Disabilities | 77
Chapter 11—Inclusive Society: Identifying and Overcoming Barriers | 79
Chapter 12—Navigating Disability Disclosure in the Workplace | 83
Chapter 13—Inclusive Growth: The Role of People with Disabilities in Modern Business | 87

Part 3: Recovery, Rehabilitation, and Caregiving
Chapter 14—The Importance of Early Intervention | 93
    Section 14.1—Act Early: The Power of Early Intervention | 94
    Section 14.2—Early Intervention in Childhood Hearing Loss | 96
    Section 14.3—Early Hearing Detection | 98
Chapter 15—Communication Strategies and Technologies | 103
    Section 15.1—Communication Techniques for Individuals with Hearing Loss | 104
    Section 15.2—Developing Communication Skills in Children with Hearing Loss | 107
    Section 15.3—American Sign Language | 109
    Section 15.4—Assistive Devices for Enhanced Communication | 111
    Section 15.5—Hearing Aids | 114
    Section 15.6—Cochlear Implants | 116
Chapter 16—Speech-Language Pathology | 121
    Section 16.1—Roles and Responsibilities of Speech-Language Pathologists | 122
    Section 16.2—Speech Therapy for Veterans | 124
    Section 16.3—Speech-Language Therapy for Autism Spectrum Disorder | 126
Chapter 17—Overcoming Learning Challenges | 129
Chapter 18—Tips for Caregivers of People with Disabilities | 133
Chapter 19—Speech to Speech Relay Service | 137
Chapter 20—Telecommunications Relay Service | 141

Part 4: Protections, Rights, and Benefits
Chapter 21—The Right to Effective Communication | 147
Chapter 22—Services for Students with Speech and Language Impairments | 151
Chapter 23—The Individuals with Disabilities Education Act (IDEA) | 153

Chapter 24—The Individualized Educational Plan (IEP) | 157
Chapter 25—Legal Framework for Supporting Students with
             Communication Disabilities | 161
Chapter 26—Telecommunications Access for People
             with Disabilities | 165
Chapter 27—Social Security Disability Programs | 169
       Section 27.1—Benefits for People with Disabilities | 170
       Section 27.2—Benefits for Children with Disabilities | 172
       Section 27.3—Qualifying for Social Security
                    Disability Benefits | 176

Part 5: Additional Resources

Chapter 28—Directory of Organizations Providing Support for People
             with Communication Disabilities | 181

Index | 187

Preface

ABOUT THIS BOOK
Communication disabilities affect an individual's ability to send, receive, process, or comprehend both verbal and nonverbal language. These impairments may affect hearing, speech, language, voice, and cognition, often leading to challenges in personal, social, and daily life. The causes of these disorders are varied, and in many cases, they remain unknown. According to the National Institute on Deafness and Other Communication Disorders (NIDCD), around 5 percent of children have noticeable speech disorders by first grade. Without timely intervention, communication disabilities may lead to additional mental health challenges, such as stress, depression, and social isolation.

Communication Disabilities Sourcebook, Second Edition provides a comprehensive and updated overview of the nature of communication disorders, including their causes, types, and effects on daily life. The book offers insights into recovery and rehabilitation strategies, emphasizing the importance of early intervention and the use of assistive technologies. It also covers legal rights and protections for individuals with communication disabilities and includes tips for caregivers to provide effective support. The book concludes with a directory of resources for further assistance and information.

HOW TO USE THIS BOOK
This book is divided into parts and chapters. Parts focus on broad areas of interest; chapters are devoted to single topics within a part.

Part 1: Understanding Communication Disorders explains the fundamental concepts of communication, including voice, speech, and language. It details various disorders affecting these functions, such as hearing loss, speech and language disorders, apraxia, and autism spectrum disorder, and provides statistical data on the prevalence of communication disorders in the United States.

Part 2: Promoting Inclusivity and Understanding explores how to foster an inclusive society for individuals with communication disabilities. It discusses the importance of using people-first language, navigating disability disclosure in the workplace, and breaking down barriers to communication.

Part 3: Recovery, Rehabilitation, and Caregiving focuses on addressing communication disorders through medical and social approaches. It covers early intervention, speech-language pathology, assistive technologies such as hearing aids and cochlear implants, and strategies for overcoming learning challenges. This part also offers practical advice for caregivers and provides insights into new technologies that aid communication.

Part 4: Protections, Rights, and Benefits summarizes the legal rights and protections for individuals with communication disabilities. It covers services offered under the Individuals with Disabilities Education Act (IDEA). This part also explains Individualized Education Plans (IEPs), telecommunications access for people with disabilities, and Social Security benefits available for children and adults with disabilities.

Part 5: Additional Resources includes a directory of organizations providing support for individuals with communication disabilities.

BIBLIOGRAPHIC NOTE

This volume contains documents and excerpts from publications issued by the following U.S. government agencies: ADA.gov; Centers for Disease Control and Prevention (CDC); *Eunice Kennedy Shriver* National Institute of Child Health and Human Development (NICHD); Federal Communications Commission (FCC); National Center on Birth Defects and Developmental Disabilities (NCBDDD); National Eye Institute (NEI); National Institute on Aging (NIA); National Institute on Deafness and Other Communication Disorders

(NIDCD); U.S. Bureau of Labor Statistics (BLS); U.S. Department of Education (ED); U.S. Department of Homeland Security (DHS); U.S. Department of Labor (DOL); U.S. Department of Veterans Affairs (VA); U.S. Food and Drug Administration (FDA); U.S. Social Security Administration (SSA); and USA.gov.

ABOUT THE *DISABILITY SERIES*

At the request of librarians serving the one in four Americans living with a disability, as well as those seeking information to comprehend, navigate, and manage such conditions, the *Disability Series* was developed as a specialized collection within Omnigraphics' *Health Reference Series*. Each volume comprehensively addresses a specific topic chosen based on the needs and interests of these patrons. These volumes offer authoritative health information, serving as a reliable resource for librarians to equip consumers with the necessary facts to take charge of their well-being. This empowers individuals to better understand and address health challenges faced by themselves, family members, or loved ones. Patrons in search of this information can find answers in the *Disability Series*. The *Series*, however, is not designed for diagnosing disabilities, prescribing treatments, or substituting the health-care provider-patient relationship. Anyone concerned about medical symptoms, the potential for disability, or illness is encouraged to seek professional care from an appropriate health-care provider.

If you have suggestions for future *Disability Series* topics, please email us at: custserv@infobaselearning.com.

A NOTE ABOUT SPELLING AND STYLE

Disability Series editors use *Stedman's Medical Dictionary* as an authority for questions related to the spelling of medical terms and *The Chicago Manual of Style* for questions related to grammatical structures, punctuation, and other editorial concerns. Consistent adherence is not always possible, however, because the individual volumes within the *Series* include many documents from a wide variety of different producers, and the editor's primary goal is to present material from each source as accurately as is possible. This sometimes means that information in different chapters or sections may follow other guidelines and alternate spelling authorities. For example, occasionally a copyright holder may require that eponymous terms be shown in possessive forms (Crohn's disease vs. Crohn disease) or that British spelling norms be retained (leukaemia vs. leukemia).

Part 1 | Understanding Communication Disorders

Chapter 1 | Basics of Communication

VOICE, SPEECH, AND LANGUAGE: WHAT ARE THEY?
Voice, speech, and language are unique functions that help us communicate.

What Is Voice?
"Voice" or "vocalization" is the sound humans produce when air from the lungs passes through the vocal folds in the larynx, causing them to vibrate.

What Is Speech?
"Speech" is the precisely coordinated complex muscle movements, primarily of the tongue and lips, that shape human vocalization into specific recognizable sounds.

What Is Language?
"Language" is the method by which humans communicate, share, and explain knowledge, beliefs, and behaviors. Language can be written, spoken, or expressed through signing or other gestures.[1]

UNDERSTANDING EARLY COMMUNICATION
Parents of young babies are experts at communicating with their babies long before their babies learn to talk or understand what

---

[1] "Voice, Speech, and Language: What Are They?" National Institute on Deafness and Other Communication Disorders (NIDCD), March 13, 2023. Available online. URL: www.nidcd.nih.gov/news/multimedia/voice-speech-language-what-are-they-text-version. Accessed August 1, 2024.

their parents are saying. We have all seen parents making funny faces for their babies. When a father makes a silly face, the baby might initially look surprised but then break into a wide smile or giggle and wiggle their arms or legs. Similarly, communication occurs when a mother rocks her baby after feeding, holds the baby close, and gazes into her little one's eyes.

Modes of Communication

Communication can include touch (such as rocking and holding your baby), vision (facial expressions, eye contact), gestures, and sound. Extending your arms to your infant indicates that you are about to pick them up. Other ways of communicating include smiling, laughing, hugging, kissing, and allowing your baby to keep you in sight. Your physical and visual contact with your baby reassures them that you are present and everything is safe.

Communicating with Babies with Hearing Loss

Many babies with hearing loss have some hearing (residual hearing) and can partially hear voices, especially if the person talking is very close. Speak to your baby while holding them close, but do not shout. Simply talk as you would to other babies. Your baby might be very interested in looking at faces and will begin to understand that your face and mouth are sending important messages. Therefore, frequently talk to your baby when they can see your face.

Tips for Effective Communication

- **Hold your baby close and make eye contact**. Position your baby so that they can easily see your face, helping them focus on your expressions and feel secure.
- **Minimize background noise**. This allows your baby to use their hearing to the best of their ability and helps them focus on your voice.
- **Use good lighting**. Ensure the room is well-lit but not too bright, so your baby can comfortably see your face and expressions.

- **Imitate your baby's sounds and movements.** Repeat what your baby does and wait for them to respond, fostering interactive communication.
- **Communicate during enjoyable activities.** Engage in communication while doing activities you both enjoy, making the experience pleasant and reinforcing positive interactions.
- **Allow for quiet time.** If your baby becomes fussy, give them some quiet time to avoid overwhelming them with too much communication.

These are some suggestions while you explore and begin to build communication and language with your baby. Please consult your baby's health-care professionals for more communication ideas.[2]

SPEECH AND LANGUAGE DEVELOPMENT

The first three years of life, when the brain is developing and maturing, is the most intensive period for acquiring speech and language skills. These skills develop best in a world that is rich with sounds, sights, and consistent exposure to the speech and language of others.

There appear to be critical periods for speech and language development in infants and young children when the brain is best able to absorb language. If these critical periods are allowed to pass without exposure to language, learning it will be more difficult.

What Are the Milestones for Speech and Language Development?

The first communication signs occur when an infant learns that a cry will bring food, comfort, and companionship. Newborns also begin to recognize important sounds in their environment, such as the voice of their mother or primary caretaker. As they grow, babies begin to sort out the speech sounds that compose the words of their language. By six months of age, most babies recognize the basic sounds of their native language.

---

[2] "Communication," Centers for Disease Control and Prevention (CDC), May 15, 2024. Available online. URL: www.cdc.gov/hearing-loss-children-guide/parents-guide/communicating.html. Accessed August 1, 2024.

Children vary in their development of speech and language skills. However, they follow a natural progression or timetable for mastering the skills of language. A checklist of milestones for the normal development of speech and language skills in children from birth to five years of age is included below. These milestones help doctors and other health professionals determine if a child is on track or if they may need extra help. Sometimes a delay may be caused by hearing loss, while other times it may be due to a speech or language disorder.

What Is the Difference between a Speech Disorder and a Language Disorder?

Children with trouble understanding what others say (receptive language) or difficulty sharing their thoughts (expressive language) may have a language disorder. Developmental language disorder (DLD) is a language disorder that delays the mastery of language skills. Some children with DLD may not begin to talk until their third or fourth year.

Children who have trouble producing speech sounds correctly or who hesitate or stutter when talking may have a speech disorder. Apraxia of speech (AOS) is a disorder that makes it difficult to put sounds and syllables together in the correct order to form words.

What Should You Do If Your Child's Speech or Language Appears to Be Delayed?

Talk to your child's doctor if you have any concerns. Your doctor may refer you to a speech-language pathologist (SLP), who is a health professional trained to evaluate and treat people with speech or language disorders. The SLP will discuss your child's communication and general development. They will also use special spoken tests to evaluate your child. A hearing test is often included in the evaluation because a hearing problem can affect speech and language development. Depending on the result of the evaluation, the SLP may suggest activities you can do at home to stimulate your child's development. They might also recommend a group or individual therapy or suggest further evaluation by an audiologist (a health-care professional trained to identify and measure hearing loss) or a developmental psychologist (a health-care professional with special expertise in the psychological development of infants and children).

Your Baby's Hearing and Communicative Development Checklist
Birth to Three Months
- Reacts to loud sounds.
- Calms down or smiles when spoken to.
- Recognizes your voice and calms down if crying.
- When feeding, starts or stops sucking in response to sound.
- Coos and makes pleasure sounds.
- Has a special way of crying for different needs.
- Smiles when they see you.

Four to Six Months
- Follows sounds with their eyes.
- Responds to changes in the tone of your voice.
- Notices toys that make sounds.
- Pays attention to music.
- Babbles in a speech-like way and uses many different sounds, including sounds that begin with p, b, and m.
- Laughs.
- Babbles when excited or unhappy.
- Makes gurgling sounds when alone or playing with you.

Seven Months to One Year
- Enjoys playing peek-a-boo and pat-a-cake.
- Turns and looks in the direction of sounds.
- Listens when spoken to.
- Understands words for common items such as "cup," "shoe," or "juice."
- Responds to requests ("Come here").
- Babbles using long and short groups of sounds ("tata, upup, bibibi").

- Babbles to get and keep attention.
- Communicates using gestures such as waving or holding up arms.
- Imitates different speech sounds.
- Has one or two words ("Hi," "dog," "Dada," or "Mama") by the first birthday.

One to Two Years
- Knows a few parts of the body and can point to them when asked.
- Follows simple commands ("Roll the ball") and understands simple questions ("Where's your shoe?").
- Enjoys simple stories, songs, and rhymes.
- Points to pictures, when named, in books.
- Acquires new words on a regular basis.
- Uses one- or two-word questions ("Where kitty?" or "Go bye-bye?").
- Puts two words together ("More cookie").
- Uses many different consonant sounds at the beginning of words.

Two to Three Years
- Has a word for almost everything.
- Uses two- or three-word phrases to talk about and ask for things.
- Uses k, g, f, t, d, and n sounds.
- Speaks in a way that is understood by family members and friends.
- Names objects to ask for them or to direct attention to them.

Three to Four Years
- Hears you when you call from another room.
- Hears the television or radio at the same sound level as other family members.
- Answers simple "Who?" "What?" "Where?" and "Why?" questions.
- Talks about activities at daycare, preschool, or friends' homes.

- Uses sentences with four or more words.
- Speaks easily without having to repeat syllables or words.

Four to Five Years
- Pays attention to a short story and answers simple questions about it.
- Hears and understands most of what is said at home and in school.
- Uses sentences that give many details.
- Tells stories that stay on topic.
- Communicates easily with other children and adults.
- Says most sounds correctly except for a few (l, s, r, v, z, ch, sh, and th).
- Uses rhyming words.
- Names some letters and numbers.
- Uses adult grammar.[3]

---

[3] "Speech and Language Developmental Milestones," National Institute on Deafness and Other Communication Disorders (NIDCD), October 13, 2022. Available online. URL: www.nidcd.nih.gov/health/speech-and-language. Accessed August 7, 2024.

Chapter 2 | The Importance of Communication and Its Disorders

IMPORTANCE OF COMMUNICATION

Communication allows us to participate in society and is a defining characteristic of what it is to be human. Other organisms clearly communicate; however, in no other species does it appear that communication—specifically the use of language in communication—is as highly developed as in humans nor as central to an organism's function and identity. Communication impairments that involve voice, speech, or language often limit a person's ability to participate in society, whether the activity is educational, occupational, or social. In addition, because effective communication is needed to get aid in life-threatening situations, loss of communication can put people at risk for compromised physical safety and survival.

BRAIN AND SENSORY INTEGRATION IN COMMUNICATION

Human communication requires the brain to integrate complex sensory signals collected by the peripheral organs and to produce neural signals to coordinate the muscles involved in speaking and signing language. Human communication systems also rely on the sensory functions of the peripheral organs responsible for hearing, balance, taste, and smell, located in the middle and inner ear, nose, mouth, and throat. They also involve vision (used for sign language and visible speech) and the development of abstract linguistic representations and memory mechanisms, located centrally in the brain. Additionally, communication systems rely on the motor functions of the hands and arms (for sign language and co-speech gestures) and on the peripheral organs of speech production, which include the diaphragm, airway, vocal folds, tongue, lips, and other oral structures.

VULNERABILITIES IN LANGUAGE ACQUISITION

The interplay between central and peripheral signals, genetics, and the environment makes language acquisition a vulnerable process. The causes of many voice, speech, and language disorders and the path to treatment are often uncertain. Gaps hinder the ability of researchers to develop effective treatment in evidence for age-appropriate clinical goals, targets of intervention, and expected change trajectories. Hence, researchers are only beginning to understand the developmental course of voice, speech, and language markers during childhood that serve as guides for clinical interventions suited to particular levels of development. There is a need for more research on communication restrictions associated with diseases and disorders most commonly occurring in adults.

ALTERNATIVE MODES OF COMMUNICATION

While spoken language is the primary way people communicate, it is not the only way. The symbolic nature of language allows us to attribute meaning through not only the voice, speech, language, and hearing but also visual-manual modes of communication, most notably the use of sign languages and augmentative and alternative communication (AAC) systems.

DEVELOPMENTAL COMMUNICATION DISORDERS

According to data from the National Health Interview Survey (NHIS), 2012, nearly 8 percent of U.S. children aged 3–17 have had a communication disorder. In children, delayed speech and language acquisition or impairment are very often significant predictors of future academic, social, vocational, and adaptive outcomes. These impairments also tend to run in families, with converging evidence of genetic effects. Many communication disorders, such as specific language impairment (SLI) and stuttering, first become apparent when a child begins to acquire speech and language. Other developmental disorders may also include communication difficulties associated with autism spectrum disorder (ASD), fragile X syndrome, or cerebral palsy (CP). One of the hallmarks of ASD is a diminished ability to communicate effectively—particularly in the expression and reception of language.

LANGUAGE AND LITERACY

Hearing loss in infancy and childhood may give rise to difficulties in acquiring spoken and written language skills. Children who are deaf are at greater risk for delays in learning to read. Children with typical hearing who have specific language impairments often have reading difficulties upon entry into school. Low proficiency in reading and writing limits job opportunities and economic success. Reading, writing, and communication skills are improving as the National Institute on Deafness and Other Communication Disorders (NIDCD) completes more research on effective ways to teach and address literacy issues in these populations.

VOICE AND VOICE DISORDERS

About 7.5 million people in the United States have trouble using their voices. Vocal fold tissue, a complex biological structure needed for optimal voice production, is susceptible to damage from daily insults from environmental pollutants or acid reflux. Such damage may compromise vocal fold integrity over time. Laryngeal disorders can cause a significant societal burden due to work-related disability, loss of productivity, and direct health-care costs (estimated at $11 billion annually).

COMMUNICATION DISORDERS AND NEURODEGENERATIVE DISORDERS

Stroke is a leading cause of adult disability in the United States. A significant proportion of stroke survivors have communication disorders, such as poststroke difficulty in using language (aphasia) or difficulty in articulating words (dysarthria) caused by brain injury. Additionally, neurodegenerative disorders, such as Parkinson disease (PD) or amyotrophic lateral sclerosis (ALS), and injury can lead to impairments in planning and executing motor speech production, such as in apraxia or dysarthria. These types of communication disorders are a strong predictor of increased isolation and poor quality of life (QOL).[1]

---

[1] "NIDCD Strategic Plan 2017–2021," National Institute on Deafness and Other Communication Disorders (NIDCD), January 2017. Available online. URL: www.nidcd.nih.gov/sites/default/files/Documents/NIDCD-StrategicPlan2017-508.pdf. Accessed August 7, 2024.

Chapter 3 | Statistics on Communication Disorders

VOICE, SPEECH, LANGUAGE, AND SWALLOWING STATISTICS
- Nearly 1 in 12 (7.7%) U.S. children aged 3–17 has had a disorder related to voice, speech, language, or swallowing in the past 12 months.
- Among children who have a voice, speech, language, or swallowing disorder, 34 percent of those aged 3–10 have multiple communication or swallowing disorders, while 25.4 percent of those aged 11–17 have multiple disorders.
- Boys aged 3–17 are more likely than girls to have a voice, speech, language, or swallowing disorder (9.6% compared to 5.7%).
- The prevalence of voice, speech, language, or swallowing disorders is highest among children aged 3–6 (11.0%), compared to children aged 7–10 (9.3%) and children aged 11–17 (4.9%).
- Nearly 1 in 10, or 9.6 percent, of Black children (aged 3–17) has a voice, speech, language, or swallowing disorder, compared to 7.8 percent of white children and 6.9 percent of Hispanic children.
- More than half (55.2%) of U.S. children aged 3–17 with a voice, speech, language, or swallowing disorder received intervention services in the past year. White children (aged 3–17) with a voice, speech, language, or swallowing disorder are more likely to have received intervention services in the past 12 months, compared to Hispanic and Black children, at 60.1, 47.3, and 45.8 percent, respectively.

- Boys (aged 3–17) with a voice, speech, language, or swallowing disorder are more likely than girls to receive intervention services, at 59.4 and 47.8 percent, respectively.
- Among children aged 3–17 who have a voice, speech, language, or swallowing disorder, those with speech or language problems, 67.6 and 66.8 percent, respectively, are more likely to receive intervention services compared to those who have a voice disorder (22.8%) or swallowing problems (12.7%).

VOICE STATISTICS

- An estimated 17.9 million U.S. adults aged 18 or older, or 7.6 percent, report having had a problem with their voice in the past 12 months. Approximately, 9.4 million (4.0%) adults report having a problem using their voice that lasted one week or longer during the last 12 months.
- 1.4 percent of U.S. children have a voice disorder that lasted for a week or longer during the past 12 months.
- Spasmodic dysphonia, a voice disorder caused by involuntary movements of one or more muscles of the larynx (voice box), can affect anyone. The first signs of this disorder are found most often in people aged 30–50. More women than men appear to be affected.

SPEECH STATISTICS

- 5 percent of U.S. children aged 3–17 have a speech disorder that lasted for a week or longer during the past 12 months.
- The prevalence of speech sound disorders (namely, articulation disorders or phonological disorders) in young children is 8–9 percent. By the first grade, roughly 5 percent of children have noticeable speech disorders, including stuttering, speech sound disorders, and dysarthria; the majority of these speech disorders have no known cause.
- More than 3 million Americans (about 1%) stutter. Stuttering can affect individuals of all ages but occurs most frequently in young children between the ages of two and six. Boys are two to three times more likely than girls to stutter.

Although most children who stutter outgrow the condition while young, as many as one in four will continue to stutter for the rest of their lives, a condition known as "persistent developmental stuttering."

LANGUAGE STATISTICS

- Developmental language disorder (also called "specific language impairment") has a prevalence of 7 percent or approximately 1 in 14 children.
- Approximately, 2 percent of children with a language disorder also have an existing medical condition (e.g., autism, intellectual disability).
- 3.3 percent of U.S. children aged 3–17 have a language disorder that lasted for a week or longer during the past 12 months.
- Research suggests that the first six months of life are the most crucial to a child's development of language skills. For a person to become fully competent in any language, exposure must begin as early as possible, preferably before school age.
- Anyone can acquire aphasia (a loss of the ability to use or understand language), but most people who have aphasia are in their middle to late years. Men and women are equally affected. Nearly 180,000 Americans acquire the disorder each year. About 2 million people in the United States currently have aphasia.

SWALLOWING STATISTICS

- 0.9 percent of U.S. children aged 3–17 have a swallowing disorder that lasted for a week or longer during the past 12 months.[1]

---

[1] "Quick Statistics about Voice, Speech, Language," National Institute on Deafness and Other Communication Disorders (NIDCD), March 4, 2024. Available online. URL: www.nidcd.nih.gov/health/statistics/quick-statistics-voice-speech-language. Accessed August 8, 2024.

Chapter 4 | Disorders of Voice, Speech, and Language

Chapter Contents
Section 4.1—Voice Health and Care 20
Section 4.2—Hoarseness 23
Section 4.3—Spasmodic Dysphonia.....................................27
Section 4.4—Vocal Fold Paralysis 30
Section 4.5—Apraxia of Speech...32
Section 4.6—Stuttering..36
Section 4.7—Developmental Language Disorder 40

Section 4.1 | Voice Health and Care

WHAT IS A VOICE?

The sound of your voice is produced by the vibration of the vocal folds, which are two bands of smooth muscle tissue that are positioned opposite each other in the larynx. The larynx is located between the base of the tongue and the top of the trachea, which is the passageway to the lungs.

When you are not speaking, the vocal folds are open so that you can breathe. When it is time to speak, however, the brain orchestrates a series of events. The vocal folds snap together while air from the lungs blows past, making them vibrate. The vibrations produce sound waves that travel through the throat, nose, and mouth, which act as resonating cavities to modulate the sound. The quality of your voice—its pitch, volume, and tone—is determined by the size and shape of the vocal folds and the resonating cavities. This is why people's voices sound so different.

Many people use their voices for their work. Singers, teachers, doctors, lawyers, nurses, salespeople, and public speakers are among those who make great demands on their voices. This puts them at risk for developing voice problems. An estimated 17.9 million adults in the United States report problems with their voice. Some of these disorders can be avoided by taking care of your voice.

HOW DO YOU KNOW WHEN YOUR VOICE IS NOT HEALTHY?

If you answer "yes" to any of the following questions, you may have a voice problem:
- Has your voice become hoarse or raspy?
- Have you lost your ability to hit some high notes when singing?
- Does your voice suddenly sound deeper?
- Does your throat often feel raw, achy, or strained?
- Has it become an effort to talk?
- Do you find yourself repeatedly clearing your throat?

If you think you have a voice problem, consult a doctor to determine the underlying cause. A doctor who specializes in diseases or

Disorders of Voice, Speech, and Language | 21

disorders of the ears, nose, and throat and who can best diagnose a voice disorder is an otolaryngologist, sometimes called an "ENT." Your otolaryngologist may refer you to a speech-language pathologist (SLP). A SLP can help you improve the way you use your voice.

WHAT CAUSES VOICE PROBLEMS?
Causes of voice problems include:
- upper respiratory infections (URIs)
- inflammation caused by gastroesophageal reflux disease (GERD; sometimes called "acid reflux" or "heartburn")
- vocal misuse and overuse
- growths on the vocal folds, such as vocal nodules or laryngeal papillomatosis
- cancer of the larynx
- neurological diseases (such as spasmodic dysphonia or vocal fold paralysis)
- psychological trauma

Most voice problems can be reversed by treating the underlying cause or through a range of behavioral and surgical treatments.

HEALTHY HABITS TO TAKE CARE OF YOUR VOICE
Staying Hydrated
- **Drink plenty of water, especially when exercising.**
- **Balance caffeinated beverages and alcohol with water.** If you drink caffeinated beverages or alcohol, balance your intake with plenty of water.
- **Take vocal naps.** Rest your voice throughout the day.
- **Use a humidifier in your home; this is especially important in winter or dry climates.** 30 percent humidity is recommended.
- **Avoid or limit the use of medications that may dry out the vocal folds, including some common cold and allergy medications.** If you have voice problems, ask your doctor which medications would be safest for you to use.

Maintaining a Healthy Lifestyle and Diet
- **Do not smoke and avoid secondhand smoke.** Smoke irritates the vocal folds. Also, cancer of the vocal folds is seen most often in individuals who smoke.
- **Avoid eating spicy foods.** Spicy foods can cause stomach acid to move into the throat or esophagus, causing heartburn or GERD.
- **Include plenty of whole grains, fruits, and vegetables in your diet.** These foods contain vitamins A, E, and C and help keep the mucus membranes that line the throat healthy.
- **Wash your hands often to prevent getting a cold or the flu.**
- **Get enough rest.** Physical fatigue has a negative effect on voice.
- **Exercise regularly.** Exercise increases stamina and muscle tone. This helps provide good posture and breathing, which are necessary for proper speaking.
- **If you have persistent heartburn or GERD, talk to your doctor about diet changes or medications that can help reduce flare-ups.**
- **Avoid mouthwash or gargles that contain alcohol or irritating chemicals.**
- **Avoid using mouthwash to treat persistent bad breath.** Halitosis (bad breath) may be the result of a problem that mouthwash cannot cure, such as low-grade infections in the nose, sinuses, tonsils, gums, or lungs or gastric acid reflux from the stomach.

Using Your Voice Wisely
- **Try not to overuse your voice.** Avoid speaking or singing when your voice is hoarse or tired.
- **Rest your voice when you are sick.** Illness puts extra stress on your voice.
- **Avoid using the extremes of your vocal range, such as screaming or whispering.** Talking too loudly and too softly can both stress your voice.

- **Practice good breathing techniques when singing or talking.** Support your voice with deep breaths from the chest and do not rely on your throat alone. Singers and speakers are often taught exercises that improve this kind of breath control. Talking from the throat, without supporting breath, puts a great strain on the voice.
- **Avoid cradling the phone when talking.** Cradling the phone between the head and shoulder for extended periods of time can cause muscle tension in the neck.
- **Consider using a microphone when appropriate.** In relatively static environments such as exhibit areas, classrooms, or exercise rooms, a lightweight microphone, and an amplifier-speaker system can be very helpful.
- **Avoid talking in noisy places.** Trying to talk above noise causes strain on the voice.
- **Consider voice therapy.** A SLP who is experienced in treating voice problems can teach you how to use your voice in a healthy way.[1]

Section 4.2 | Hoarseness

WHAT IS HOARSENESS?
If you are hoarse, your voice will sound breathy, raspy, or strained or will be softer in volume or lower in pitch. Your throat might feel scratchy. Hoarseness is often a symptom of problems in the vocal folds of the larynx.

HOW DOES OUR VOICE WORK?
The sound of our voice is produced by the vibration of the vocal folds, which are two bands of smooth muscle tissue that are positioned

---

[1] "Taking Care of Your Voice," National Institute on Deafness and Other Communication Disorders (NIDCD), April 15, 2021. Available online. URL: www.nidcd.nih.gov/health/taking-care-your-voice. Accessed August 8, 2023.

opposite each other in the larynx. The larynx is located between the base of the tongue and the top of the trachea, which is the passageway to the lungs.

When we are not speaking, the vocal folds are open so that we can breathe. When it is time to speak, however, the brain orchestrates a series of events. The vocal folds snap together while air from the lungs blows past, making them vibrate. The vibrations produce sound waves that travel through the throat, nose, and mouth, which act as resonating cavities to modulate the sound. The quality of our voice—its pitch, volume, and tone—is determined by the size and shape of the vocal folds and the resonating cavities. This is why people's voices sound so different.

Individual variations in our voices are the result of how much tension we put on our vocal folds. For example, relaxing the vocal folds makes a voice deeper; tensing them makes a voice higher.

WHEN SHOULD YOU SEE THE DOCTOR IF YOUR VOICE IS HOARSE?

You should see your doctor if your voice has been hoarse for more than three weeks, especially if you have not had a cold or the flu. You should also see a doctor if you are coughing up blood or if you have difficulty swallowing, feel a lump in your neck, experience pain when speaking or swallowing, have difficulty breathing, or lose your voice completely for more than a few days.

HOW WILL YOUR DOCTOR DIAGNOSE WHAT IS WRONG?

Your doctor will ask you about your health history and how long you have been hoarse. Depending on your symptoms and general health, your doctor may send you to an otolaryngologist (a doctor who specializes in diseases of the ears, nose, and throat). An otolaryngologist will usually use an endoscope (a flexible, lighted tube designed for looking at the larynx) to get a better view of the vocal folds. In some cases, your doctor might recommend special tests to evaluate voice irregularities or vocal airflow.

WHAT ARE SOME OF THE DISORDERS THAT CAUSE HOARSENESS, AND HOW ARE THEY TREATED?

Hoarseness can have several possible causes and treatments, including the following:

Laryngitis

This is one of the most common causes of hoarseness. It can be due to temporary swelling of the vocal folds from a cold, an upper respiratory infection (URI), or allergies. Your doctor will treat laryngitis according to its cause. If it is due to a cold or URI, your doctor might recommend rest, fluids, and nonprescription pain relievers. Allergies might be treated similarly, with the addition of over-the-counter (OTC) allergy medicines.

Misusing or Overusing Your Voice

Cheering at sporting events, speaking loudly in noisy situations, talking for too long without resting your voice, singing loudly, or speaking with a voice that is too high or too low can cause temporary hoarseness. Resting, reducing voice use, and drinking lots of water should help relieve hoarseness from misuse or overuse. Sometimes, people whose jobs depend on their voices—such as teachers, singers, or public speakers—develop hoarseness that will not go away. If you use your voice for a living and you regularly experience hoarseness, your doctor might suggest seeing a speech-language pathologist (SLP) for voice therapy. In voice therapy, you will be given vocal exercises and tips for avoiding hoarseness by changing the ways in which you use your voice.

Gastroesophageal Reflux Disease

Gastroesophageal reflux disease (GERD)—commonly called "heartburn"—can cause hoarseness when stomach acid rises up to the throat and irritates the tissues. Usually, hoarseness caused by GERD is worse in the morning and improves throughout the day. In some people, the stomach acid rises all the way up to the throat and larynx and irritates the vocal folds. This is called "laryngopharyngeal reflux" (LPR). LPR can happen during the day or night. Some people will have no heartburn with LPR, but they may feel as if they constantly have to cough to clear their throat, and they may become hoarse. GERD and LPR are treated with dietary modifications and medications that reduce stomach acid.

Vocal Nodules, Polyps, and Cysts

These are benign (noncancerous) growths within or along the vocal folds. Vocal nodules are sometimes called "singer's nodes" because they are a frequent problem among professional singers. They form in pairs on opposite sides of the vocal folds as the result of too much pressure or friction, such as the way a callus forms on the foot from a shoe that is too tight. A vocal polyp typically occurs only on one side of the vocal fold. A vocal cyst is a hard mass of tissue encased in a membrane sac inside the vocal fold. The most common treatments for nodules, polyps, and cysts are voice rest, voice therapy, and surgery to remove the tissue.

Vocal Fold Hemorrhage

This occurs when a blood vessel on the surface of the vocal fold ruptures and the tissues fill with blood. If you lose your voice suddenly during strenuous vocal use (such as yelling), you may have a vocal fold hemorrhage. Sometimes, a vocal fold hemorrhage will cause hoarseness to develop quickly over a short amount of time and only affect your singing but not your speaking voice. Vocal fold hemorrhage must be treated immediately with total voice rest and a trip to the doctor.

Vocal Fold Paralysis

This is a voice disorder that occurs when one or both of the vocal folds do not open or close properly. It can be caused by injury to the head, neck, or chest; lung or thyroid cancer; tumors of the skull base, neck, or chest; or infection (e.g., Lyme disease). People with certain neurological conditions, such as multiple sclerosis (MS) or Parkinson disease (PD), or those who have sustained a stroke may experience vocal fold paralysis. In many cases, however, the cause is unknown. Vocal fold paralysis is treated with voice therapy and, in some cases, surgery.

Neurological Diseases and Disorders

Neurological conditions that affect areas of the brain that control muscles in the throat or larynx can also cause hoarseness.

Hoarseness is sometimes a symptom of PD or a stroke. Spasmodic dysphonia is a rare neurological disease that causes hoarseness and can also affect breathing. Treatment in these cases will depend upon the type of disease or disorder.

Other Causes

Thyroid problems and injury to the larynx can cause hoarseness. Hoarseness may sometimes be a symptom of laryngeal cancer, which is why it is so important to see your doctor if you are hoarse for more than three weeks. Hoarseness is also the most common symptom of a disease called "recurrent respiratory papillomatosis" (RRP), or "laryngeal papillomatosis," which causes noncancerous tumors to grow in the larynx and other air passages leading from the nose and mouth into the lungs.[1]

Section 4.3 | Spasmodic Dysphonia

WHAT IS SPASMODIC DYSPHONIA?

Spasmodic dysphonia, or laryngeal dystonia, is a disorder affecting the voice muscles in the larynx, also called the "voice box." When you speak, air from your lungs is pushed between two elastic structures—called "vocal folds"—causing them to vibrate and produce your voice. In spasmodic dysphonia, the muscles inside the vocal folds spasm, making sudden, involuntary movements and interfering with vocal fold vibrations. Spasmodic dysphonia may occur alongside other forms of dystonia that cause repeated spasms in other parts of the body, including the eyes, face, jaw, lips, tongue, neck, arms, or legs.

Spasmodic dysphonia causes voice breaks during speech, making the voice sound tight, strained, or breathy. In some individuals, these breaks can occur as frequently as once every few sentences, significantly affecting their ability to communicate. In more severe cases, spasms may occur on every word, making a person's speech

---

[1] "Hoarseness," National Institute on Deafness and Other Communication Disorders (NIDCD), March 6, 2017. Available online. URL: www.nidcd.nih.gov/health/hoarseness. Accessed August 8, 2023.

very difficult to understand. Some people with spasmodic dysphonia may also have vocal tremor—a shaking of the larynx and vocal folds that causes the voice to tremble.

Spasmodic dysphonia is a chronic condition that persists throughout a person's life. It may develop suddenly with severe voice symptoms present from the onset of the disorder, or it may begin with mild symptoms and occur only occasionally before worsening and becoming more frequent over time.

Spasmodic dysphonia is a rare disorder. It can affect anyone, but the first signs most often occur in people between the ages of 30 and 50. It affects more women than men.

WHAT ARE THE TYPES OF SPASMODIC DYSPHONIA?

Spasmodic dysphonia can be classified into the following three types:

Adductor Spasmodic Dysphonia

This is the most common form of spasmodic dysphonia. In this disorder, spasms cause the vocal folds to slam together and stiffen. These spasms make it difficult for the vocal folds to vibrate and produce sounds. The voice of someone with adductor spasmodic dysphonia may sound strained and strangled. The person's speech may be choppy, with words cut off or difficult to start because of muscle spasms. The spasms are usually absent—and the voice sounds normal—while laughing, crying, or whispering. Stress often makes the muscle spasms more severe.

Abductor Spasmodic Dysphonia

This form is less common. In this disorder, spasms cause the vocal folds to remain open. The vocal folds cannot vibrate when they are open too far. The open position also allows air to escape from the lungs during speech. As a result, the voice often sounds weak and breathy. As with adductor spasmodic dysphonia, the spasms are often absent during activities such as laughing, crying, or whispering.

Mixed Spasmodic Dysphonia

This type is a combination of the two types mentioned earlier and is very rare. It features both the muscle behaviors of the opening and closing of the vocal folds.

WHAT CAUSES SPASMODIC DYSPHONIA?

Spasmodic dysphonia is thought to be caused by abnormal functioning in an area of the brain called the "basal ganglia," which helps coordinate muscle movements throughout the body. Research has found abnormalities in other regions of the brain associated with spasmodic dysphonia, including areas of the cerebral cortex that control commands to muscles and coordinate these commands with incoming sensory information.

In some cases, spasmodic dysphonia may run in families. Although a specific gene for spasmodic dysphonia has not yet been identified, a mutation in a gene that causes other forms of dystonia has also been associated with spasmodic dysphonia.

HOW IS SPASMODIC DYSPHONIA DIAGNOSED?

Diagnosis of spasmodic dysphonia can be challenging because the symptoms often resemble those of other voice disorders. Diagnosis usually follows examination by a team, including the following:

- **Otolaryngologist.** A doctor who specializes in diseases of the ear, nose, throat, head, and neck will pass a small lighted tube through the nose and into the back of the throat—a procedure called "fiberoptic nasolaryngoscopy"—to evaluate vocal fold anatomy and movements during speech and other activities of the larynx.
- **Speech-language pathologist (SLP).** A health professional trained to evaluate and treat voice, speech, and language disorders will assess voice symptoms.
- **Neurologist.** A doctor who specializes in nervous system disorders will evaluate for signs in the brain of dystonia and other movement disorders.

WHAT TREATMENT IS AVAILABLE FOR SPASMODIC DYSPHONIA?

Currently, there is no cure for spasmodic dysphonia, but treatment can help reduce its symptoms. The most common treatment is the injection of very small amounts of botulinum toxin directly into the affected muscles of the larynx. Botulinum toxin injections are more effective with adductor spasmodic dysphonia than with abductor spasmodic dysphonia and do not help in every case.

Behavioral therapy (voice therapy) may reduce symptoms in mild cases. Voice therapy may work along with botulinum toxin injections to reduce voice strain. Some people may also benefit from psychological counseling to help them accept and live with their voice problems.

Augmentative and assistive devices can help some people with spasmodic dysphonia communicate more easily. Some devices can help amplify a person's voice, whether in person or over the phone. Computer software and tablet or smartphone apps can translate text into synthetic speech.

A physician can explain the potential outcomes, risks, and benefits of surgical treatment and can help manage expectations.[1]

Section 4.4 | Vocal Fold Paralysis

WHAT IS VOCAL FOLD PARALYSIS?

Vocal fold paralysis, also known as "vocal cord paralysis," is a voice disorder that occurs when one or both vocal folds do not open or close properly. Single vocal fold paralysis is a common disorder, but paralysis of both vocal folds is rare and can be life-threatening.

If you have vocal fold paralysis, the paralyzed fold or folds may remain open, leaving the air passages and lungs unprotected. You could experience difficulty swallowing, or food or liquids could accidentally enter the trachea and lungs, causing serious health problems.

WHAT CAUSES VOCAL FOLD PARALYSIS?

Vocal fold paralysis may be caused by injury to the head, neck, or chest; lung or thyroid cancer; tumors of the skull base, neck, or chest; or infection, such as Lyme disease. People with certain neurological conditions, such as multiple sclerosis (MS) or Parkinson disease (PD)

---

[1] "Spasmodic Dysphonia," National Institute on Deafness and Other Communication Disorders (NIDCD), June 18, 2020. Available online. URL: www.nidcd.nih.gov/health/spasmodic-dysphonia. Accessed August 8, 2024.

or those who have sustained a stroke, may experience vocal fold paralysis. In many cases, however, the cause is unknown.

WHAT ARE THE SYMPTOMS OF VOCAL FOLD PARALYSIS?

Symptoms of vocal fold paralysis include changes in the voice, such as hoarseness or a breathy voice; difficulties with breathing, such as shortness of breath or noisy breathing; and swallowing problems, such as choking or coughing when you eat because food is accidentally entering the windpipe instead of the esophagus (the muscular tube that connects the throat to the stomach). Changes in voice quality, such as loss of volume or pitch, may also occur. Damage to both vocal folds, although rare, usually causes serious problems with breathing.

HOW IS VOCAL FOLD PARALYSIS DIAGNOSED?

An otolaryngologist usually diagnoses vocal fold paralysis—a doctor specializing in ear, nose, and throat disorders. The otolaryngologist will inquire about your symptoms and when the problems began to help determine their cause. He or she will also listen to your voice to identify breathiness or hoarseness. Using an endoscope, a tube with a light at the end, your doctor will look directly into the throat at the vocal folds. Some doctors also use a procedure called "laryngeal electromyography," which measures the electrical impulses of the nerves in the larynx, to better understand the areas of paralysis.

HOW IS VOCAL FOLD PARALYSIS TREATED?

The most common treatments for vocal fold paralysis are voice therapy and surgery. Some people's voices naturally recover sometime during the first year after diagnosis, so doctors often delay surgery for at least a year. During this time, your doctor will likely refer you to a speech-language pathologist (SLP) for voice therapy, which may involve exercises to strengthen the vocal folds or improve breath control while speaking. You might also learn to use your voice in a different way, such as by speaking more slowly, opening your mouth wider when speaking, or using specific vocal techniques to reduce strain and improve clarity. Several surgical procedures are available, depending on whether one or both of your vocal folds are paralyzed. The most common procedure is to change the position of the vocal fold. These may involve inserting a structural implant or stitches to reposition the laryngeal cartilage and bring the vocal folds closer together. These procedures usually result in a stronger voice. Surgery is followed by additional voice therapy to help fine-tune the voice.

When both vocal folds are paralyzed, a tracheotomy may be required to assist breathing. In a tracheotomy, an incision is made in the front of the neck, and a breathing tube is inserted through an opening, called a "stoma," into the trachea. Breathing then occurs through the tube rather than through the nose and mouth. Following surgery, therapy with an SLP helps you learn how to use the voice and how to properly care for the breathing tube.[1]

Section 4.5 | Apraxia of Speech

WHAT IS APRAXIA OF SPEECH?

Apraxia of speech (AOS)—also known as "acquired apraxia of speech," "verbal apraxia," or "childhood apraxia of speech" (CAS) when diagnosed in children—is a speech sound disorder. Someone with AOS has trouble saying what they want to say correctly and consistently. Apraxia of speech is a neurological disorder that affects the brain pathways involved in planning the sequence of movements necessary for producing speech. The brain knows what it wants to say but cannot properly plan and sequence the required speech sound movements.

Apraxia of speech is not caused by weakness or paralysis of the speech muscles (the muscles of the jaw, tongue, or lips). Weakness or paralysis of the speech muscles results in a separate speech disorder, known as "dysarthria." Some people have both dysarthria and AOS, which can complicate the diagnosis of the two conditions.

The severity of AOS varies from person to person. It can be so mild that it causes trouble with only a few speech sounds or with

---

[1] "Vocal Fold Paralysis," National Institute on Deafness and Other Communication Disorders (NIDCD), March 6, 2017. Available online. URL: www.nidcd.nih.gov/health/vocal-fold-paralysis. Accessed August 8, 2024.

the pronunciation of words that have many syllables. In the most severe cases, someone with AOS might not be able to communicate effectively by speaking and may need the help of alternative communication methods.

WHAT ARE THE TYPES AND CAUSES OF APRAXIA OF SPEECH?

The following are the two main types of AOS:

- **Acquired AOS**. Although it most typically occurs in adults, it can affect someone at any age. It is caused by damage to the parts of the brain that are involved in speaking and involves the loss or impairment of existing speech abilities. It may result from a stroke, head injury, tumor, or other illness affecting the brain. Acquired AOS may occur together with other conditions that are caused by damage to the nervous system. One of these is dysarthria, as mentioned earlier. Another is "aphasia," which is a language disorder.
- **Childhood AOS**. This condition is present from birth and is also known as "developmental apraxia of speech," "developmental verbal apraxia," or "articulatory apraxia." Childhood AOS is not the same as developmental delays in speech, in which a child follows the typical path of speech development but does so more slowly than is typical. The causes of childhood AOS are not well understood. Imaging and other studies have not been able to find evidence of brain damage or differences in the brain structure of children with AOS. Children with AOS often have family members who have a history of communication disorders or learning disabilities. This observation and recent research findings suggest that genetic factors may play a role in the disorder. Childhood AOS appears to affect more boys than girls.

WHAT ARE THE SYMPTOMS OF APRAXIA OF SPEECH?

People with either form of AOS may exhibit a number of different speech characteristics or symptoms:

- **Distorting sounds**. People with AOS may have difficulty pronouncing words correctly. Sounds, especially vowels,

are often distorted. Because the speaker may not place the speech structures (e.g., tongue, jaw) quite in the right place, the sound comes out wrong. Longer or more complex words are usually harder to say than shorter or simpler words. Sound substitutions might also occur when AOS is accompanied by aphasia.
- **Making inconsistent errors in speech**. For example, someone with AOS may say a difficult word correctly but then have trouble repeating it or may be able to say a particular sound one day and have trouble with the same sound the next day.
- **Groping for sounds**. People with AOS often appear to be groping for the right sound or word and may try saying a word several times before they say it correctly.
- **Making errors in tone, stress, or rhythm**. Another common characteristic of AOS is the incorrect use of prosody. Prosody is the rhythm and inflection of speech that we use to help express meaning. Someone who has trouble with prosody might use equal stress, segment syllables in a word, omit syllables in words and phrases, or pause inappropriately while speaking.

Children with AOS generally understand language much better than they can use it. Some children with the disorder may also have other speech problems, expressive language problems, or motor skill problems.

HOW IS APRAXIA OF SPEECH DIAGNOSED?

Professionals known as "speech-language pathologists" (SLPs) play a key role in diagnosing and treating AOS. Because there is no single symptom or test that can be used to diagnose AOS, the professional making the diagnosis generally looks for the presence of several of a group of symptoms, including those described earlier. Ruling out other conditions, such as muscle weakness or language production problems (e.g., aphasia), can help with the diagnostic process.

In formal testing for both acquired and childhood AOS, a SLP may ask the patient to perform speech tasks such as repeating a particular word several times or repeating a list of words of increasing length (e.g., love, loving, lovingly). For acquired AOS, a SLP may also examine the patient's ability to converse, read, write, and perform nonspeech movements. To diagnose childhood AOS, parents and professionals may need to observe a child's speech over a period of time.

HOW IS APRAXIA OF SPEECH TREATED?

In some cases, people with acquired AOS recover some or all of their speech abilities on their own. This is called "spontaneous recovery."

Children with AOS will not outgrow the problem on their own. They also do not acquire the basics of speech just by being around other children, such as in a classroom. Therefore, speech-language therapy is necessary for children with AOS as well as for people with acquired AOS who do not spontaneously recover all of their speech abilities.

Speech-language pathologists use different approaches to treat AOS, and no single approach has been proven to be the most effective. Therapy is tailored to the individual and is designed to treat other speech or language problems that may occur together with AOS. Frequent, intensive, one-on-one speech-language therapy sessions are needed for both children and adults with AOS (The repetitive exercises and personal attention needed to improve AOS are difficult to deliver in group therapy.). Children with severe AOS may need intensive speech-language therapy for years, in parallel with normal schooling, to obtain adequate speech abilities.

Some adults and children will make more progress during treatment than others. Support and encouragement from family members and friends and extra practice in the home environment are important.[1]

---

[1] "Apraxia of Speech," National Institute on Deafness and Other Communication Disorders (NIDCD), October 31, 2017. Available online. URL: www.nidcd.nih.gov/health/apraxia-speech. Accessed August 8, 2024.

Section 4.6 | Stuttering

WHAT IS STUTTERING?

Stuttering is a speech disorder characterized by the repetition of sounds, syllables, or words, prolongation of sounds, and interruptions in speech known as "blocks." An individual who stutters knows exactly what they would like to say but has trouble producing a normal flow of speech. These speech disruptions may be accompanied by struggle behaviors, such as rapid eye blinks or tremors of the lips. Stuttering can make it difficult to communicate with others, often affecting a person's quality of life (QOL) and interpersonal relationships. It can also negatively influence job performance and opportunities, and treatment can be costly.

Symptoms of stuttering can vary significantly throughout a person's day. Generally, speaking before a group or talking on the telephone may exacerbate a person's stuttering, while singing, reading, or speaking in unison may temporarily alleviate it.

Stuttering is sometimes referred to as "stammering" and, more broadly, as "disfluent speech."

WHO IS AFFECTED BY STUTTERING?

Approximately, 3 million Americans stutter. It affects people of all ages but occurs most often in children between the ages of two and six as they develop their language skills. About 5–10 percent of all children will experience stuttering for some period, lasting from a few weeks to several years. Boys are two to three times as likely to stutter as girls, and this gender difference increases with age; the number of boys who continue to stutter is three to four times larger than the number of girls. Most children outgrow stuttering, with about 75 percent recovering. For the remaining 25 percent, stuttering can persist as a lifelong communication disorder.

HOW IS SPEECH NORMALLY PRODUCED?

We make speech sounds through a series of precisely coordinated muscle movements involving breathing, phonation (voice production), and articulation (movement of the throat, palate, tongue, and lips).

The brain controls these muscle movements, which are monitored through our senses of hearing and touch.

WHAT ARE THE CAUSES AND TYPES OF STUTTERING?
The precise mechanisms that cause stuttering are not fully understood. Stuttering is commonly grouped into two types: developmental and neurogenic.

Developmental Stuttering
Developmental stuttering occurs in young children as they are still learning speech and language skills. It is the most common form of stuttering. Some scientists and clinicians believe it occurs when children's speech and language abilities cannot meet their verbal demands. Most believe developmental stuttering results from complex interactions of multiple factors. Brain imaging studies have shown consistent differences in those who stutter compared to their non-stuttering peers. It may also run in families, and genetic factors are believed to play a role. Since 2010, researchers at the National Institute on Deafness and Other Communication Disorders (NIDCD) have identified four genes where mutations are associated with stuttering.

Neurogenic Stuttering
Neurogenic stuttering may occur after a stroke, head trauma, or other brain injuries. In cases of neurogenic stuttering, the brain struggles to coordinate the various brain regions involved in speaking, resulting in problems with producing clear, fluent speech.

Historically, all stuttering was thought to be psychogenic, caused by emotional trauma; however, we now know that psychogenic stuttering is rare.

HOW IS STUTTERING DIAGNOSED?
A speech-language pathologist (SLP), trained to test and treat individuals with voice, speech, and language disorders, usually diagnoses stuttering. This specialist will consider various factors, including the child's case history, an analysis of the stuttering behaviors, and

an evaluation of the child's speech and language abilities and how stuttering affects their lives.

When evaluating a young child for stuttering, a SLP will try to determine whether the child is likely to continue stuttering or outgrow it. Factors considered include the family history of stuttering, whether the stuttering has persisted for six months or longer, and whether the child exhibits other speech or language problems.

HOW IS STUTTERING TREATED?

Although no cure for stuttering exists, various treatments are available. The type of treatment depends on the person's age, communication goals, and other factors. It is important to work with a SLP to determine the best treatment options.

Therapy for Children

For very young children, early treatment may prevent developmental stuttering from becoming a lifelong issue. Certain strategies can help children improve their speech fluency and develop positive attitudes toward communication. Health professionals generally recommend evaluation for children who have stuttered for three to six months, exhibit struggle behaviors associated with stuttering, or have a family history of stuttering or related communication disorders. Some researchers recommend evaluating a child every three months to assess whether the stuttering is increasing or decreasing. Treatment often involves educating parents on supporting their child's fluent speech production. Parents may be encouraged to do the following:

- Provide a relaxed home environment that allows many opportunities for the child to speak, including setting aside time to talk to one another, especially when the child is excited and has a lot to say.
- Listen attentively when the child speaks and focus on the content of the message rather than on how it is said, refraining from interrupting.
- Speak in a slightly slowed and relaxed manner, which can help reduce the time pressures the child may be experiencing.

- Listen attentively and wait for the child to say the intended word, without completing their sentences, helping them understand that successful communication can occur even when stuttering happens.
- Discuss stuttering openly and honestly if the child brings up the subject, ensuring the child understands that some disruptions are normal.

Stuttering Therapy

Therapies for teens and adults who stutter focus on learning ways to minimize stuttering, such as speaking more slowly, regulating breathing, or gradually progressing from single-syllable responses to longer words and more complex sentences. These therapies also address the anxiety individuals may feel in certain speaking situations.

Drug Therapy

The U.S. Food and Drug Administration (FDA) has not approved any drugs specifically for stuttering treatment. However, some drugs approved for other conditions—such as epilepsy, anxiety, or depression—have been used off-label for stuttering. These drugs often have side effects that make long-term use challenging.

Electronic Devices

Some individuals who stutter use electronic devices to help control fluency. For example, one type of device fits into the ear canal, similar to a hearing aid, and replays a slightly altered version of the wearer's voice into the ear, making it sound as if they are speaking in unison with another person. These devices may improve fluency in a relatively short period, but additional research is needed to assess their long-term effectiveness and usability in real-world situations.

Self-Help Groups

Many find that combining self-study with therapy leads to the greatest success. Self-help groups offer resources and support, helping individuals who stutter face the challenges associated with the condition.[1]

Section 4.7 | Developmental Language Disorder

WHAT IS DEVELOPMENTAL LANGUAGE DISORDER?

Developmental language disorder (DLD) is a communication disorder that interferes with the ability to learn, understand, and use language. These language difficulties are not explained by other conditions, such as hearing loss or autism, or by extenuating circumstances, such as limited exposure to language. DLD can affect a child's ability to speak, listen, read, and write. Previously referred to as "specific language impairment," "language delay," or "developmental dysphasia," DLD is one of the most common developmental disorders, affecting approximately 1 in 14 children in kindergarten. Its effect persists into adulthood.

WHAT CAUSES DEVELOPMENTAL LANGUAGE DISORDER?

Developmental language disorder (DLD) is a neurodevelopmental disorder caused by complex interactions between genes and the environment that alter brain development. The exact causes of the brain differences that lead to DLD remain unknown.

Neurodevelopmental disorders often run in families. Children with DLD are more likely than those without DLD to have parents and siblings who have also experienced language development difficulties and delays. In fact, 50–70 percent of children with DLD have at least one family member with the disorder. Additionally, other potentially related neurodevelopmental disorders, such as dyslexia or autism, are more common among the family members of a child with DLD.

Learning more than one language simultaneously does not cause DLD. The disorder can affect both multilingual children and children

---

[1] "Stuttering," National Institute on Deafness and Other Communication Disorders (NIDCD), March 6, 2017. Available online. URL: www.nidcd.nih.gov/health/stuttering. Accessed August 8, 2024.

who speak only one language. For multilingual children, DLD will affect all languages spoken by the child. Importantly, learning multiple languages is not detrimental to a child with DLD. A multilingual child with DLD will not struggle more than a monolingual child with DLD.

WHAT ARE THE SYMPTOMS OF DEVELOPMENTAL LANGUAGE DISORDER?

A child with DLD often has a history of being a late talker, reaching spoken language milestones later than peers. Although some late talkers eventually catch up with their peers, children with DLD have persistent language difficulties.

Younger children with DLD may:
- be late to form words into sentences
- struggle to learn new words and engage in conversation
- have difficulty following directions, not due to stubbornness, but because they do not fully comprehend the spoken words
- make frequent grammatical errors when speaking

Symptoms common in older children and adults with DLD include:
- limited use of complex sentences
- difficulty finding the right words
- challenges with understanding figurative language
- reading difficulties
- disorganized storytelling and writing
- frequent grammatical and spelling errors

HOW IS DEVELOPMENTAL LANGUAGE DISORDER DIAGNOSED?

If a doctor, teacher, or parent suspects that a child has DLD, a speech-language pathologist (SLP)—a professional trained to assess and treat individuals with speech or language problems—can evaluate the child's language skills. The type of evaluation depends on the

child's age and the concerns that prompted the evaluation. Generally, an evaluation includes:
- direct observation of the child
- interviews and questionnaires completed by parents and/or teachers
- assessments of the child's learning ability
- standardized tests of current language performance

These tools allow the SLP to compare the child's language skills to those of same-age peers, identify specific difficulties, and plan potential treatment targets.

WHAT ARE THE TREATMENTS AVAILABLE FOR DEVELOPMENTAL LANGUAGE DISORDER?

Treatment services for DLD are typically provided or overseen by a licensed SLP. Treatment may occur in homes, schools, university programs for speech-language pathology, private clinics, or outpatient hospital settings.

Identifying and treating children with DLD early is ideal, but individuals can benefit from treatment regardless of when it begins. Treatment depends on the age and needs of the individual. Starting treatment early can help young children to:
- acquire missing elements of grammar
- expand their understanding and use of words
- develop social communication skills

For school-age children, treatment may focus on understanding instruction in the classroom, including helping with issues such as:
- following directions
- understanding the meaning of words that teachers use
- organizing information
- improving speaking, reading, and writing skills[1]

---

[1] "Developmental Language Disorder," National Institute on Deafness and Other Communication Disorders (NIDCD), May 8, 2023. Available online. URL: www.nidcd.nih.gov/health/developmental-language-disorder. Accessed August 8, 2024.

Chapter 5 | Specific Language Impairment

WHAT IS SPECIFIC LANGUAGE IMPAIRMENT?
Specific language impairment (SLI) is a communication disorder that disrupts the development of language skills in children who do not have hearing loss. SLI can affect a child's speaking, listening, reading, and writing abilities. It is also known as "developmental language disorder" (DLD), language delay, or developmental dysphasia. SLI is one of the most common developmental disorders, affecting approximately 7–10 percent of children in kindergarten. Among those children with language impairment, about 2–3 percent also have an existing medical condition and/or intellectual disability. The effects of SLI usually persist into adulthood.

WHAT CAUSES SPECIFIC LANGUAGE IMPAIRMENT?
The cause of SLI is unknown, but research suggests a strong genetic link. Children with SLI are more likely than those without SLI to have parents and siblings who have also experienced difficulties and delays in speaking. In fact, 50–70 percent of children with SLI have at least one family member with the disorder. Learning more than one language at a time does not cause SLI, and the disorder can affect both multilingual children and children who speak only one language.

WHAT ARE THE SYMPTOMS OF SPECIFIC LANGUAGE IMPAIRMENT?
A child with SLI often has a history of being a late talker, reaching spoken language milestones later than peers. Preschool-aged children with SLI may:
- be late to form words into sentences
- struggle to learn new words and engage in conversation

- have difficulty following directions, not because they are stubborn but because they do not fully understand the spoken words
- make frequent grammatical errors when speaking

Although some late talkers eventually catch up with their peers, children with SLI have persistent language difficulties. Symptoms common in older children and adults with SLI include:
- limited use of complex sentences
- difficulty finding the right words
- challenges with understanding figurative language
- reading difficulties
- disorganized storytelling and writing
- frequent grammatical and spelling errors

HOW IS SPECIFIC LANGUAGE IMPAIRMENT DIAGNOSED?

If a doctor, teacher, or parent suspects that a child has SLI, a speech-language pathologist (SLP)—a professional trained to assess and treat people with speech or language problems—can evaluate the child's language skills. The type of evaluation depends on the child's age and the concerns that led to the evaluation. Generally, an evaluation includes:
- direct observation of the child
- interviews and questionnaires completed by parents and/or teachers
- assessments of the child's learning ability
- standardized tests of current language performance

These tools allow the SLP to compare the child's language skills to those of same-age peers, identify specific difficulties, and plan for potential treatment targets.

WHAT ARE THE TREATMENTS AVAILABLE FOR SPECIFIC LANGUAGE IMPAIRMENT?

Treatment services for SLI are typically provided or overseen by a licensed SLP. Treatment may be provided in homes, schools, university programs for speech-language pathology, private clinics, or outpatient hospitals. Identifying and treating children with SLI early

Specific Language Impairment | 45

in life is ideal, but individuals can benefit from treatment regardless of when it begins. Treatment depends on the age and needs of the person. Starting treatment early can help young children:
- acquire missing elements of grammar
- expand their understanding and use of words
- develop social communication skills

For school-age children, treatment may focus on understanding instruction in the classroom, including helping with issues such as:
- following directions
- understanding the meaning of the words that teachers use
- organizing information
- improving speaking, reading, and writing skills[1]

---

[1] "Specific Language Impairment," National Institute on Deafness and Other Communication Disorders (NIDCD), July 15, 2019. Available online. URL: www.nidcd.nih.gov/sites/default/files/Documents/health/voice/specific-language-impairment.pdf. Accessed August 8, 2024.

Chapter 6 | Sensory Impairments Affecting Communication

Chapter Contents
Section 6.1—Hearing Disorders..48
Section 6.2—Low Vision...51

Section 6.1 | Hearing Disorders

Hearing loss is a common problem caused by loud noise, aging, disease, and genetic variations. About one-third of older adults experience hearing loss, and the likelihood of developing hearing loss increases with age. People with hearing loss may find it challenging to have conversations with friends and family. They may also have difficulty understanding a doctor's advice, responding to warnings, and hearing doorbells and alarms.

Some people may not want to admit they have trouble hearing, but ignoring or leaving hearing problems untreated can make them worse. If you suspect you have a hearing problem, consult your doctor. Treatments that can help include hearing aids, special training, certain medications, and surgery.

SIGNS OF HEARING LOSS

Some people may have a hearing problem without realizing it. You should see your doctor if you:
- have trouble understanding what people are saying over the telephone
- find it hard to follow conversations when two or more people are talking
- often ask people to repeat what they are saying
- need to turn up the TV volume so loud that others complain
- have difficulty understanding speech because of background noise
- think that others seem to mumble
- cannot understand what is being said when children and people with higher-pitched voices speak to you

TYPES OF HEARING LOSS

Hearing loss varies in severity. It can range from mild loss, where a person misses certain high-pitched sounds, to total hearing loss.

Sudden Hearing Loss

Sudden deafness, also known as "sudden sensorineural hearing loss," is an unexplained rapid loss of hearing that can occur all at once or over a few days. It should be treated as a medical emergency. If you or someone you know experiences sudden hearing loss, it is important to seek medical attention immediately to prevent potential long-term damage and identify the underlying cause.

Age-Related Hearing Loss

Age-related hearing loss, referred to as "presbycusis," develops gradually as a person ages. It seems to run in families and may result from changes in the inner ear and auditory nerve, which relays signals from the ear to the brain. Presbycusis may make it difficult for a person to tolerate loud sounds or to understand what others are saying.

Age-related hearing loss usually affects both ears equally. Because the loss is gradual, people with presbycusis may not realize they have lost some of their hearing ability.

Tinnitus

Tinnitus is also common among older people. It is typically described as ringing in the ears, but it can also sound like roaring, clicking, hissing, or buzzing. Tinnitus can come and go and may be heard in one or both ears, either loudly or softly. It is sometimes the first sign of hearing loss in older adults and can accompany any type of hearing loss.

Tinnitus is a symptom, not a disease. Something as simple as a piece of earwax blocking the ear canal can cause tinnitus. It can also be a sign of other health conditions, such as high blood pressure (HBP) or allergies, or it may be a side effect of certain medications.

CAUSES OF HEARING LOSS

Loud noise is one of the most common causes of hearing loss. Noise from lawnmowers, snow blowers, or loud music can damage the inner ear, leading to permanent hearing loss. Loud noise also contributes to tinnitus. You can prevent most noise-related hearing loss by turning down the sound on your devices, moving away from loud noise, or using earplugs or other ear protection.

Earwax or fluid buildup can also cause hearing loss by blocking sounds that are carried from the eardrum to the inner ear. If wax blockage is a problem, your doctor may suggest mild treatments to soften earwax.

A ruptured eardrum can also cause hearing loss. The eardrum can be damaged by infection, pressure, or by inserting objects into the ear, including cotton-tipped swabs. See your doctor if you experience ear pain or fluid drainage from an ear.

Health conditions common in older people, such as diabetes or HBP, can contribute to hearing loss. Ear infections caused by viruses and bacteria (also known as "otitis media" (OM)), a heart condition, stroke, brain injury, or a tumor may also affect your hearing.

Hearing loss can also result from taking certain medications that can damage the inner ear, sometimes permanently. These medications may be used to treat serious infections, cancer, or heart disease. They also include some antibiotics and even aspirin at certain dosages. If you notice a problem while taking a medication, consult your doctor.

Genetic variations can also cause hearing loss. Not all inherited forms of hearing loss are evident at birth; some may appear later in life. For example, otosclerosis, thought to be a hereditary disease, involves the abnormal growth of bone that prevents structures within the ear from functioning properly.

HOW TO COPE WITH HEARING LOSS

If you notice signs of hearing loss, talk with your doctor. If you have trouble hearing, do the following:

- Let your family and friends know you have a hearing problem.
- Ask people to face you and to speak louder and more clearly. Ask them to repeat themselves or reword what they are saying.
- Pay attention to what is being said and to facial expressions or gestures.
- Let the person talking know if you do not understand what was said.
- Find a good location to listen. Place yourself between the speaker and sources of noise or look for quieter places to talk.

The most important thing you can do if you think you have a hearing problem is to seek professional advice. Your family doctor may be able to diagnose and treat your hearing problem. Alternatively, your doctor may refer you to other experts, such as an otolaryngologist (ear, nose, and throat doctor) or an audiologist (health professional who can identify and measure hearing loss).[1]

Section 6.2 | Low Vision

WHAT IS LOW VISION?

Low vision is a condition that makes it difficult to perform everyday activities. It cannot be corrected with glasses, contact lenses, or other standard treatments such as medication or surgery.

You may have low vision if you cannot see well enough to do things such as:

- **Read.** Difficulty reading books, newspapers, or digital screens.
- **Drive.** Inability to drive safely or legally.
- **Recognize people's faces.** Challenges in identifying familiar faces.
- **Tell colors apart.** Difficulty distinguishing between colors.
- **See your television or computer screen clearly.** Blurred or unclear view of screens.

TYPES OF LOW VISION

The type of low vision you have depends on the disease or condition that caused it. The most common types of low vision include:

- **Central vision loss.** Inability to see things in the center of your vision.
- **Peripheral vision loss.** Difficulty seeing things out of the corners of your eyes.

---

[1] National Institute on Aging (NIA), "Hearing Loss: A Common Problem for Older Adults," National Institutes of Health (NIH), January 19, 2023. Available online. URL: www.nia.nih.gov/health/hearing-and-hearing-loss/hearing-loss-common-problem-older-adults#cope. Accessed August 8, 2024.

- **Night blindness.** Difficulty seeing in low light or darkness.
- **Blurry or hazy vision.** A general lack of clarity in vision.

CAUSES OF LOW VISION

Many eye conditions can cause low vision. The most common causes include:
- **Age-related macular degeneration (AMD).** A condition that affects the central part of the retina.
- **Cataracts.** Clouding of the eye's lens.
- **Diabetic retinopathy (DR).** Vision loss caused by diabetes.
- **Glaucoma.** A group of eye conditions that damage the optic nerve.

Low vision is more common in older adults because many of the diseases that can cause it are more prevalent in this age group. However, aging alone does not cause low vision. Eye and brain injuries, as well as certain genetic disorders, can also cause low vision.

HOW YOUR DOCTOR WILL CHECK FOR LOW VISION

Your doctor can check for low vision as part of a dilated eye exam, which is simple and painless. During the exam, your doctor will ask you to read letters that are up close and far away and will check whether you can see things in the center and at the edges of your vision.

They will give you eye drops to dilate (widen) your pupils and check for other eye problems, including conditions that could cause low vision.

TREATMENT FOR LOW VISION

Unfortunately, low vision is usually permanent. Eyeglasses, medication, and surgery typically cannot cure low vision, but sometimes they can improve vision, help you perform everyday activities more easily, or prevent further vision loss.

Treatment options will depend on the specific eye condition that caused your low vision. Consult your doctor to learn about any treatments that could improve your vision or help protect your remaining vision.

Sensory Impairments Affecting Communication | 53

TIPS FOR MAXIMIZING VISION IF YOU HAVE LOW VISION
If you have low vision, there are ways to maximize your vision and continue enjoying the activities you love.

For Minor Vision Loss
- Use brighter lights at home or work to improve visibility.
- Wear anti-glare sunglasses to reduce discomfort from bright light.
- Use a magnifying lens for reading and other close-up activities.

For Significant Vision Loss
If your vision loss interferes with daily activities, consider vision rehabilitation. A specialist can help you adapt to your vision loss, offering:
- training on how to use a magnifying device for reading
- guidance for setting up your home to facilitate movement and safety
- resources to help you cope with vision loss[1]

---

[1] "At a Glance: Low Vision," National Eye Institute (NEI), November 15, 2023. Available online. URL: www.nei.nih.gov/learn-about-eye-health/eye-conditions-and-diseases/low-vision. Accessed August 8, 2024.

Chapter 7 | Central Auditory Processing Disorder

Children who have difficulty using information they hear in academic and social situations may have central auditory processing disorder (CAPD), more recently termed "auditory processing disorder" (APD). These children typically can hear information but have difficulty attending to, storing, locating, retrieving, and/or clarifying that information to make it useful for academic and social purposes. This can negatively affect both language acquisition and academic performance.

WHAT IS CENTRAL AUDITORY PROCESSING?
When the ears detect sound, the auditory stimulus travels through the structures of the ears, or the peripheral auditory system, to the central auditory nervous system, which extends from the brain stem to the temporal lobes of the cerebral cortex. The auditory stimulus travels along the neural pathways where it is "processed," allowing the listener to determine the direction from which the sound comes, identify the type of sound, separate the sound from background noise, and interpret the sound. The listener builds upon what is heard by storing, retrieving, or clarifying the auditory information to make it functionally useful.

WHAT IS A DISORDER OF AUDITORY PROCESSING?
Auditory processing disorder is an impaired ability to attend to, discriminate, remember, recognize, or comprehend information presented auditorily in individuals who typically exhibit normal intelligence and normal hearing. This definition has been expanded to include how peripheral hearing loss may contribute to auditory processing deficits. Auditory processing difficulties

become more pronounced in challenging listening situations, such as noisy backgrounds or poor acoustic environments, great distances from the speaker, speakers with fast speaking rates, or speakers with foreign accents.

HOW IS AUDITORY PROCESSING DISORDER DIAGNOSED?

Given the complexity of auditory processing disorders, it is important to involve a multidisciplinary team, including psychologists, physicians, teachers, parents, and, of course, audiologists and speech-language pathologists (SLPs). Audiologists diagnose the presence of APD (hearing and processing problems), and SLPs evaluate a child's perception of speech and receptive-expressive language use. Other team members conduct additional assessments to determine a child's educational strengths and weaknesses. Checklists that ask teachers and parents to observe the child's auditory behaviors may be used to determine the need for an APD evaluation. The parent's description of the child's auditory behavior at home is an especially important contribution to diagnosing APD.

WHAT DOES THE AUDIOLOGIST DO?

The audiologist assesses the peripheral and central auditory systems using a battery of tests, which may include both electrophysiological and behavioral tests. Peripheral hearing tests determine if the child has a hearing loss and, if so, the degree to which the loss is a factor in the child's learning problems. Assessment of the central auditory system evaluates the child's ability to respond under different conditions of auditory signal distortion and competition. It is based on the assumption that a child with an intact auditory system can tolerate mild distortions of speech and still understand it, while a child with APD will encounter difficulty when the auditory system is stressed by signal distortion and competing messages. The test results allow the audiologist to identify strengths and weaknesses in the child's auditory system that can be used to develop educational and remedial intervention strategies.

HOW SHOULD TEST RESULTS BE INTERPRETED?

As with any kind of evaluation, test results should be interpreted with caution. The effects of neurological maturation may influence test results for children under the age of 12 years. A true diagnosis of APD cannot be determined until that time. However, there are much younger children whose auditory behaviors, language, and academic characteristics indicate that APD is a strong possibility, and even without a formal diagnosis, these children would benefit from intervention. Remediation should address their strengths and areas of need based on available speech-language and psychoeducational testing.[1]

---

[1] "Auditory Processing Disorders: An Overview," U.S. Department of Education (ED), December 2002. Available online. URL: https://files.eric.ed.gov/fulltext/ED474303.pdf. Accessed August 8, 2024.

Chapter 8 | Other Disorders Affecting Communication

Chapter Contents
Section 8.1—Aphasia...60
Section 8.2—Orofacial Clefts..62
Section 8.3—Autism Spectrum Disorder 65
Section 8.4—Effects of Low Birth Weight on Communication
　　　　　　　and Development 67

Section 8.1 | Aphasia

WHAT IS APHASIA?

Aphasia is a disorder resulting from damage to portions of the brain responsible for language. For most people, these areas are on the left side of the brain. Aphasia usually occurs suddenly, often following a stroke or head injury, but it may also develop slowly as a result of a brain tumor or a progressive neurological disease. The disorder impairs the expression and understanding of language as well as reading and writing. Aphasia may co-occur with speech disorders, such as dysarthria or apraxia of speech (AOS), which also result from brain damage.

WHO CAN ACQUIRE APHASIA?

Most people with aphasia are middle-aged or older, but anyone can acquire it, including young children. About 1 million people in the United States currently have aphasia, and nearly 180,000 Americans acquire it each year, according to the National Aphasia Association.

WHAT CAUSES APHASIA?

Aphasia is caused by damage to one or more of the language areas of the brain. Most often, the cause of the brain injury is a stroke.

WHAT ARE THE DIFFERENT TYPES OF APHASIA?

There are two broad categories of aphasia: fluent and nonfluent, and there are several types within these groups.

Damage to the temporal lobe of the brain may result in Wernicke aphasia, the most common type of fluent aphasia. People with Wernicke aphasia may speak in long, complete sentences that have no meaning, adding unnecessary words and even creating made-up words.

- For example, someone with Wernicke aphasia may say, "You know that smoodle pinkered and that I want to get him round and take care of him like you want before."

The most common type of nonfluent aphasia is Broca aphasia. People with Broca aphasia have damage that primarily affects the frontal lobe of the brain. They often have right-sided weakness or paralysis of the arm and leg because the frontal lobe is also important for motor movements. People with Broca aphasia may understand speech and know what they want to say, but they frequently speak in short phrases that are produced with great effort. They often omit small words, such as "is," "and," and "the."

- For example, a person with Broca aphasia may say, "Walk dog," meaning, "I will take the dog for a walk," or "book book two table" for "There are two books on the table." People with Broca aphasia typically understand the speech of others fairly well. Because of this, they are often aware of their difficulties and can become easily frustrated.

HOW IS APHASIA DIAGNOSED?

Aphasia is usually first recognized by the physician who treats the person for his or her brain injury. Most individuals will undergo a magnetic resonance imaging (MRI) or computed tomography (CT) scan to confirm the presence of a brain injury and to identify its precise location. The physician also typically tests the person's ability to understand and produce language, such as following commands, answering questions, naming objects, and carrying on a conversation.

HOW IS APHASIA TREATED?

Following a brain injury, tremendous changes occur in the brain that help it recover. As a result, people with aphasia often see dramatic improvements in their language and communication abilities in the first few months, even without treatment. However, in many cases, some aphasia remains following this initial recovery period. In these instances, speech-language therapy is used to help patients regain their ability to communicate.

Aphasia therapy aims to improve a person's communication ability by helping him or her use remaining language abilities, restore language abilities as much as possible, and learn other ways of communicating, such as gestures, pictures, or electronic devices. Individual therapy focuses on the specific needs of the person, while group therapy offers the opportunity to use new communication skills in a small-group setting.

Family involvement is often a crucial component of aphasia treatment because it enables family members to learn the best way to communicate with their loved ones.

Family members are encouraged to:
- participate in therapy sessions, if possible
- simplify language by using short, uncomplicated sentences
- repeat the content words or write down keywords to clarify meaning as needed
- maintain a natural conversational manner appropriate for an adult
- minimize distractions, such as a loud radio or TV, whenever possible
- include the person with aphasia in conversations
- ask for and value the opinion of the person with aphasia, especially regarding family matters
- encourage any type of communication, whether it is speech, gesture, pointing, or drawing
- avoid correcting the person's speech
- allow the person plenty of time to talk
- help the person become involved outside the home (Seek out support groups, such as stroke clubs.)[1]

Section 8.2 | Orofacial Clefts

UNDERSTANDING OROFACIAL CLEFTS
Cleft Lip

The lip forms between the fourth and seventh weeks of pregnancy. During development, body tissue and special cells from each side of the head grow toward the center of the face. They join together to form facial features like the lips and mouth.

---

[1] "Aphasia," National Institute on Deafness and Other Communication Disorders (NIDCD), March 6, 2017. Available online. URL: www.nidcd.nih.gov/health/aphasia. Accessed August 8, 2024.

Other Disorders Affecting Communication | 63

A cleft lip occurs when the tissue making up the upper lip does not join completely before birth, leaving an opening (see Figure 8.1). The opening can be small or extend through the lip into the nose.

A cleft lip can occur on one or both sides of the lip or in the middle of the lip. Children with a cleft lip may also have a cleft palate.

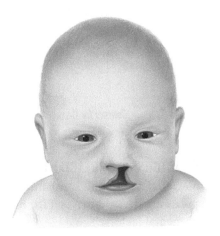

Figure 8.1. Cleft Lip
Centers for Disease Control and Prevention (CDC)

Cleft Palate

The roof of the mouth (palate) forms between the sixth and ninth weeks of pregnancy. A cleft palate occurs when the tissue that makes up the palate does not completely join (see Figure 8.2). For some babies, both the front and back parts of the palate are open. For others, only part of the palate is open.

Together, these birth defects are called "orofacial clefts." If the orofacial clefts are not surgically repaired, children with these conditions may experience problems with feeding and speaking clearly. They may also have ear infections, hearing problems, or issues with their teeth.

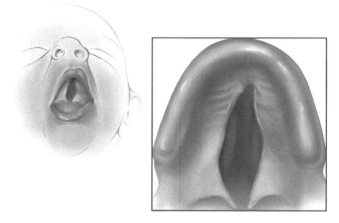

Figure 8.2. Cleft Palate
Centers for Disease Control and Prevention (CDC)

CAUSES AND RISK FACTORS OF OROFACIAL CLEFTS

The causes of orofacial clefts among most infants are unknown. Cleft lip and cleft palate are thought to result from a combination of genetic and environmental factors.

Some factors that increase the risk of having a baby with an orofacial cleft are:
- smoking during pregnancy
- having type 1 or 2 diabetes before pregnancy
- use of certain epilepsy medications during pregnancy

DIAGNOSIS OF OROFACIAL CLEFTS

Orofacial clefts, especially cleft lip, can often be diagnosed during pregnancy through a routine ultrasound. They can also be diagnosed after the baby is born. Certain types of cleft palate (e.g., submucous cleft palate and bifid uvula) might not be diagnosed until later in life.

TREATMENT FOR OROFACIAL CLEFTS

Services and treatment for children with orofacial clefts can vary depending on the severity of the cleft, the child's age and needs, and the presence of associated syndromes or other birth defects.

Surgery to repair a cleft lip usually occurs in the first few months of life. It is recommended within the first 12 months of life. Surgery to repair a cleft palate is recommended within the first 18 months of life, or earlier if possible. Many children will need additional surgical procedures as they grow older.

Surgical repair can help restore function to the lips and mouth and may improve breathing, hearing, speech, and language development. Children born with orofacial clefts may also need special dental or orthodontic care or speech therapy.

With treatment, most children with orofacial clefts do well and lead healthy lives. Some children may experience self-esteem issues if they are concerned with visible differences between themselves and others. Parent-to-parent support groups can be valuable for families of babies with orofacial clefts.[1]

Section 8.3 | Autism Spectrum Disorder

Autism spectrum disorder (ASD) is a developmental disability that can cause significant social, communication, and behavioral challenges. The term "spectrum" refers to the wide range of symptoms, skills, and levels of impairment that people with ASD can have.

ASD affects people in different ways and can range from mild to severe. While individuals with ASD share some common symptoms, such as difficulties with social interaction, there are differences in the onset of symptoms, their severity, the number of symptoms, and the presence of other conditions. The symptoms and their severity can change over time.

The behavioral signs of ASD often appear early in development, with many children showing symptoms between 12 and 18 months of age, or even earlier.

---

[1] "Cleft Lip/Cleft Palate," Centers for Disease Control and Prevention (CDC), May 16, 2024. Available online. URL: www.cdc.gov/birth-defects/about/cleft-lip-cleft-palate.html. Accessed August 9, 2024.

WHO IS AFFECTED BY AUTISM SPECTRUM DISORDER?

Autism spectrum disorder affects people of every race, ethnic group, and socioeconomic background. It is four times more common among boys than among girls. The Centers for Disease Control and Prevention (CDC) estimates that about 1 in every 54 children in the United States has been identified as having ASD.

HOW DOES AUTISM SPECTRUM DISORDER AFFECT COMMUNICATION?

Children with ASD are often self-absorbed and seem to exist in a private world, with a limited ability to successfully communicate and interact with others. They may have difficulty developing language skills and understanding what others say to them. Additionally, they often struggle with nonverbal communication, such as hand gestures, eye contact, and facial expressions.

The ability of children with ASD to communicate and use language depends on their intellectual and social development. Some children with ASD may not be able to communicate using speech or language and may have very limited speaking skills. Others may have rich vocabularies and be able to talk about specific subjects in great detail. However, many have problems with the meaning and rhythm of words and sentences, and may also be unable to understand body language and different vocal tones. These difficulties, taken together, affect the ability of children with ASD to interact with others, especially peers.

Below are some patterns of language use and behaviors often found in children with ASD:

- repetitive or rigid language
- narrow interests and exceptional abilities
- uneven language development
- poor nonverbal conversation skills

HOW ARE THE SPEECH AND LANGUAGE PROBLEMS OF AUTISM SPECTRUM DISORDER TREATED?

If a doctor suspects a child has ASD or another developmental disability, they will typically refer the child to a variety of specialists, including a speech-language pathologist (SLP). This health professional is trained to treat individuals with voice, speech, and language disorders. The SLP will perform a comprehensive evaluation of the child's ability to communicate and design an appropriate treatment program. Additionally, the SLP might refer the child for a hearing test to ensure the child's hearing is normal.

Teaching children with ASD to improve their communication skills is essential for helping them reach their full potential. There are many approaches, but the best treatment program begins early, during the preschool years, and is tailored to the child's age and interests. It should address both the child's behavior and communication skills and offer regular reinforcement of positive actions. Most children with ASD respond well to highly structured, specialized programs. Parents or primary caregivers, as well as other family members, should be involved in the treatment program so that it becomes part of the child's daily life.

For some younger children with ASD, improving speech and language skills is a realistic goal of treatment. Parents and caregivers can increase a child's chance of reaching this goal by paying attention to their language development early on. Just as toddlers learn to crawl before they walk, children first develop pre-language skills before they begin to use words. These skills include using eye contact, gestures, body movements, imitation, and babbling and other vocalizations to help them communicate. Children who lack these skills may be evaluated and treated by a SLP to prevent further developmental delays.

For slightly older children with ASD, communication training teaches basic speech and language skills, such as single words and phrases. Advanced training emphasizes how language can serve a purpose, such as learning to hold a conversation with another person, which includes staying on topic and taking turns speaking.[1]

Section 8.4 | Effects of Low Birth Weight on Communication and Development

The effects of low birth weight on communication and developmental problems extend beyond the tiniest of babies and continue

---

[1] "Autism Spectrum Disorder: Communication Problems in Children," National Institute on Deafness and Other Communication Disorders (NIDCD), April 13, 2020. Available online. URL: www.nidcd.nih.gov/health/autism-spectrum-disorder-communication-problems-children#3. Accessed August 8, 2024.

well into childhood, according to an analysis of follow-up survey data on a large, diverse group of children. The researchers found that by age 10, children in all three standard categories of low birth weight were more likely to have been diagnosed with a speech-language disorder and to have received speech-language services than children who had been born at a normal weight.

STUDY METHODOLOGY

Researchers from the National Institutes of Health (NIH), the Missouri Department of Health and Senior Services, and the University of Missouri utilized existing data from the Missouri Maternal and Infant Health Survey, which included infants born during a 16-month period between 1989 and 1991. After 10 years, parents or other caregivers of nearly 870 children from the original survey filled out an extensive questionnaire about their children, including their children's medical, educational, and social services history. The data were grouped according to the children's birth weights:

- extremely low (less than 2.2 pounds)
- very low (2.2–3.3 pounds)
- moderately low (3.3–5.5 pounds)
- normal (more than 5.5 pounds)

PREVALENCE OF SPEECH-LANGUAGE DISORDERS

Compared to children with normal birth weights, low birth weight children were two to three times more likely to have received speech-language therapy. While about 14.5 percent of children with a history of normal birth weight received speech-language therapy by age 10, about 28 percent of children with a history of moderately or very low birth weight and 39 percent of children with extremely low birth weight had received therapy.

BROADER DEVELOPMENTAL CONCERNS

Compared to children born at a normal birth weight, children across all categories of low birth weight were more likely to have used speech-language, occupational, and physical therapy services, had a higher incidence of pneumonia, and exhibited weaker motor abilities and school performance. Even moderately low birth weight children were about three times more likely to repeat a grade than their normal birth weight counterparts.

HEARING LOSS AND SPECIAL EDUCATION NEEDS

Low birth weight was not linked to hearing loss or the use of hearing aids in this study, although parents of children with extremely low birth weight reported a significantly higher rate of special seating in classrooms because of hearing problems. However, hearing problems are often underdiagnosed and underreported, and this study reports on children who were born more than a decade before universal newborn hearing screening was required in Missouri, starting in 2002.

RECOMMENDATIONS FOR SCREENING

Infants with extremely low birth weights are typically screened for health problems. The new findings suggest that thorough screening by health-care providers of all low birth weight children, even those with moderately low birth weight, may be important.[1]

---

[1] "Low Birth Weight Linked to Communication Problems in Children," National Institute on Deafness and Other Communication Disorders (NIDCD), September 25, 2019. Available online. URL: www.nidcd.nih.gov/news/2019/low-birth-weight-linked-communication-problems-children. Accessed August 8, 2024.

Part 2 | Promoting Inclusivity and Understanding

Chapter 9 | Tips for Effective Interactions with People Who Have Communication Disabilities

GENERAL TIPS
- **Engage directly with the person.** When talking to a person with a disability, look at and speak directly to that person, rather than their companion.
- **Be considerate of people's service animals.** Some people with disabilities may use a service animal. Do not pet or play with the animal, as this may unsettle the person and interrupt the animal's assistive duties.
- **Avoid assuming the preferences and needs of people with disabilities.** People with disabilities are individuals with unique preferences and needs. If you think a person may need help, ask how you may be of assistance.
- **Communicate clearly and comprehensibly.** As with all communication, an effective message is one that is spoken or written clearly and understandably. This is especially important for people with disabilities who may have difficulty obtaining or comprehending messages. Be sure to convey your message in an understandable form and in multiple ways if necessary.
- **If you do not need to know about the specific nature of someone's disability, do not ask about it.** Focus on what the person is communicating to you.

- **Relax in your conversation**. Do not be embarrassed if you use common expressions such as "See you later" or "Got to be running along" that seem to relate to the person's disability. Do not be afraid to ask questions when you are unsure of how to assist the person.

TIPS FOR A PERSON WHO HAS A HEARING DISABILITY
- **Address the person directly**. When a sign language interpreter is present, look at and speak to the person who is deaf, not the interpreter, when communicating.
- **Gain attention**. To get the attention of a person who is deaf or hard of hearing, tap them gently on the arm, wave your hand, or flicker the lights if you are in a large group.
- **Look directly at the person and speak clearly, naturally, and slowly to establish whether the person can speechread**. Not all deaf people can speechread. Those who can will rely on facial expressions and other body language to help them understand.
- **Show consideration by placing yourself under or near a light source and keeping your hands and food away from your mouth when speaking**. Shouting will not help.
- **Offer the person a means of exchanging written messages to see if that would be helpful in facilitating communication.**
- **When gathered as a group, speak one at a time**. This is especially true if sign language interpreters are being used, but it also applies to general communication.

TIPS FOR A PERSON WHO HAS A SPEECH DISABILITY
- **Listen attentively**. Keep your manner encouraging rather than correcting. Exercise patience rather than attempting to speak for a person with a speech disability.
- **Never pretend to understand if you are having difficulty doing so**. Repeat what you understand or incorporate the

person's statements into follow-up questions. The person's reactions will guide you.
- **When necessary, ask short questions that require short answers or a nod or shake of the head.**

TIPS FOR A PERSON WITH AN INTELLECTUAL OR DEVELOPMENTAL DISABILITY

- **Respect choices and decisions.** Speak directly to the person and respect their expressed preferences regarding choices or decisions.
- **Choose a quiet space.** If you are in a public area with many distractions, consider moving to a quiet or private location.
- **Be aware of the possible need to speak to the person in clear and short sentences.** Repeat your information and questions as needed. Use concrete words, visual aids, or color-based cues.
- **It may be helpful to offer assistance in completing forms or understanding written instructions, and provide extra time for decision-making.** Wait for the individual to accept the offer of assistance; do not "over-assist" or be patronizing.
- **Be patient, flexible, and supportive.** Take time to understand the individual and verify that the individual understands you.

TIPS FOR A PERSON WHO HAS A VISION DISABILITY

- **Greet the person verbally to let them know that you have approached them.** Identify yourself and others who may be with you. Speak normally while facing the person.
- **Do not grab the person's arm or cane assuming they need assistance.** Ask first if they need assistance.
- **Offer to assist the person in reaching their destination.** Offer your arm as a guide just above the elbow and describe any obstacles in the path of travel. When arriving at the destination, inform the person that they are standing in front of the chair, table, doorway, and so on. It is appropriate to

guide the person's hand to the chair or railing for additional assistance in orienting them.
- **Respect the guide dog.** If the person has a guide dog, walk on the side opposite the dog and do not touch or distract the dog at any time.
- **When conversing in a group, give a vocal cue by announcing the name of the person to whom you are speaking.**
- **Notify when moving or ending conversation.** Indicate in advance when you will be moving from one place to another, and let it be known when the conversation ends.[1]

---

[1] "A Guide to Interacting with People Who Have Disabilities," U.S. Department of Homeland Security (DHS), September 26, 2013. Available online. URL: www.dhs.gov/sites/default/files/publications/guide-interacting-with-people-who-have-disabilties_09-26-13.pdf. Accessed August 9, 2024.

Chapter 10 | The Importance of People-First Language in Discussing Disabilities

About 1 in 4 U.S. adults, or 61 million people, reports having some form of disability. Disability is part of the human experience, but sometimes people use words or phrases that are insensitive and do not promote understanding, dignity, and respect for people with disabilities. More often than not, this is unintentional, but it can still be disrespectful.

PEOPLE-FIRST LANGUAGE
People-first language is the best approach when talking to a person with a disability. If you are unsure, ask the person how they would like to be described. It is important to remember that preferences can vary.

People-first language is used to communicate appropriately and respectfully with and about an individual with a disability. This approach emphasizes the person first, not the disability. For example, when referring to a person with a disability, use phrases such as "a person who …," "a person with …," or "a person who has …"

GUIDELINES FOR USING PEOPLE-FIRST LANGUAGE
Emphasize Abilities, Not Limitations
- Use "person who uses a device to speak"; do not use "can't talk" or "mute."
- Use "person who uses a wheelchair"; do not use "confined or restricted to a wheelchair" or "wheelchair bound."
- Do not use language that suggests the lack of something.

Use Appropriate Terminology
- Use "person with a disability"; do not use "disabled" or "handicapped."
- Use "person of short stature"; do not use "midget."
- Use "person with cerebral palsy"; do not use "cerebral palsy victim."
- Use "person with epilepsy" or "person with a seizure disorder"; do not use "epileptic."
- Use "person with multiple sclerosis"; do not use "afflicted by multiple sclerosis."

Emphasize the Need for Accessibility, Not the Disability
- Use "accessible parking" or "accessible bathroom"; do not use "handicapped parking" or "handicapped bathroom."

Avoid Offensive Language
- Use "person with an intellectual, cognitive, or developmental disability"; do not use "slow, simple, moronic, defective, afflicted, special person."
- Use "person with an emotional or behavioral disability, a mental health impairment, or a psychiatric disability"; do not use "insane, crazy, psycho, maniac, nuts."
- Use "person with a physical disability"; do not use "crippled, lame, deformed, invalid, spastic."

Avoid Language That Implies Negative Stereotypes
- Use "person without a disability"; do not use "normal person" or "healthy person."
- Do not portray people with disabilities as inspirational solely because of their disability.
- Use "person who is successful, productive"; do not use "has overcome his or her disability" or "is courageous."[1]

---

[1] National Center on Birth Defects and Developmental Disabilities (NCBDDD), "Communicating with and about People with Disabilities," Centers for Disease Control and Prevention (CDC), February 1, 2022. Available online. URL: www.cdc.gov/ncbddd/disabilityandhealth/materials/factsheets/fs-communicating-with-people.html. Accessed August 7, 2024.

Chapter 11 | Inclusive Society: Identifying and Overcoming Barriers

Nearly everyone faces hardships and difficulties at one time or another. But for people with disabilities, barriers can be more frequent and have a greater effect. The World Health Organization (WHO) describes barriers as being more than just physical obstacles. Here is the WHO definition of barriers:

Factors in a person's environment that, through their absence or presence, limit functioning and create disability. These include aspects such as:
- a physical environment that is not accessible
- lack of relevant assistive technology (assistive, adaptive, and rehabilitative devices)
- negative attitudes of people toward disability
- services, systems and policies that are either nonexistent or that hinder the involvement of all people with a health condition in all areas of life

ATTITUDINAL BARRIERS

Attitudinal barriers are the most basic and contribute to other barriers. For example, some people may not be aware that difficulties in getting to or into a place can limit a person with a disability from participating in everyday life and common daily activities. Examples of attitudinal barriers include:
- **Stereotyping**. People sometimes stereotype those with disabilities, assuming their quality of life (QOL) is poor or that they are unhealthy because of their impairments.

- **Stigma, prejudice, and discrimination.** Within society, these attitudes may come from people's disability-related ideas. People may see disability as a personal tragedy, as something that needs to be cured or prevented, as a punishment for wrongdoing, or as an indication of the lack of ability to behave as expected in society.

Today, society's understanding of disability is improving as we recognize "disability" as what occurs when a person's functional needs are not addressed in their physical and social environment. By not considering disability a personal deficit or shortcoming, and instead thinking of it as a social responsibility in which all people can be supported to live independent and full lives, it becomes easier to recognize and address challenges that all people—including those with disabilities—experience.

COMMUNICATION BARRIERS

Communication barriers are experienced by people with disabilities that affect hearing, speaking, reading, writing, and/or understanding, and who use different ways to communicate than people who do not have these disabilities. Examples of communication barriers include:
- Written health promotion messages with barriers that prevent people with vision impairments from receiving the message. These include:
  - use of small print or no large-print versions of material
  - no Braille or versions for people who use screen readers
- Auditory health messages may be inaccessible to people with hearing impairments, including:
  - videos that do not include captioning
  - oral communications without accompanying manual interpretation (such as American Sign Language (ASL))
- The use of technical language, long sentences, and words with many syllables may be significant barriers to understanding for people with cognitive impairments.

PHYSICAL BARRIERS
Physical barriers are structural obstacles in natural or human-made environments that prevent or block mobility (moving around in the environment) or access. Examples of physical barriers include:
- steps and curbs that block a person with mobility impairment from entering a building or using a sidewalk
- mammography equipment that requires a woman with a mobility impairment to stand
- absence of a weight scale that accommodates wheelchairs or others who have difficulty stepping up

POLICY BARRIERS
Policy barriers are frequently related to a lack of awareness or enforcement of existing laws and regulations that require programs and activities to be accessible to people with disabilities. Examples of policy barriers include:
- denying qualified individuals with disabilities the opportunity to participate in or benefit from federally funded programs, services, or other benefits
- denying individuals with disabilities access to programs, services, benefits, or opportunities to participate as a result of physical barriers
- denying reasonable accommodations to qualified individuals with disabilities, so they can perform the essential functions of the job for which they have applied or have been hired to perform

PROGRAMMATIC BARRIERS
Programmatic barriers limit the effective delivery of a public health or health-care program for people with different types of impairments. Examples of programmatic barriers include:
- inconvenient scheduling
- lack of accessible equipment (such as mammography screening equipment)
- insufficient time set aside for medical examination and procedures

- little or no communication with patients or participants
- provider's attitudes, knowledge, and understanding of people with disabilities

SOCIAL BARRIERS

Social barriers are related to the conditions in which people are born, grow, live, learn, work, and age—or social determinants of health—that can contribute to decreased functioning among people with disabilities. Here are examples of social barriers:
- People with disabilities are far less likely to be employed. In 2017, 35.5 percent of people with disabilities, aged 18–64 years, were employed, while 76.5 percent of people without disabilities were employed, about double that of people with disabilities.
- Adults aged 18 years and older with disabilities are less likely to have completed high school compared to their peers without disabilities (22.3% compared to 10.1%).
- People with disabilities are more likely to have an income of less than $15,000 compared to people without disabilities (22.3% compared to 7.3%).
- Children with disabilities are almost four times more likely to experience violence than children without disabilities.

TRANSPORTATION BARRIERS

Transportation barriers are due to a lack of adequate transportation that interferes with a person's ability to be independent and to function in society. Examples of transportation barriers include:
- lack of access to accessible or convenient transportation for people who are not able to drive because of vision or cognitive impairments
- public transportation may be unavailable or at inconvenient distances or locations[1]

---

[1] National Center on Birth Defects and Developmental Disabilities (NCBDDD), "Common Barriers to Participation Experienced by People with Disabilities," Centers for Disease Control and Prevention (CDC), May 2, 2024. Available online. URL: www.cdc.gov/ncbddd/disabilityandhealth/disability-barriers.html. Accessed August 7, 2024.

Chapter 12 | Navigating Disability Disclosure in the Workplace

Every job seeker with a disability faces the same decision: "Should I or shouldn't I disclose my disability?" This decision may be framed differently depending on whether you have a visible or nonvisible disability. Ultimately, the decision to disclose is entirely up to you.

REASONS TO DISCLOSE YOUR DISABILITY IN THE WORKPLACE

When you leave school and enter the workforce, many aspects of your life change. Among these differences is the requirement to share information about your disability if you want your employer to provide reasonable accommodations. In school, if you had an individualized education program (IEP), as required under the Individuals with Disabilities Education Act (IDEA), information about your disability and the accommodations you needed to be followed from grade to grade. However, when you enter the workforce, the IDEA no longer applies to you. Instead, the Americans with Disabilities Act (ADA) and the Rehabilitation Act protect you from disability-related discrimination and provide for meaningful access. These laws require that qualified applicants and employees with disabilities be provided with reasonable accommodations. However, to benefit from the ADA and the Rehabilitation Act, you must disclose your disability. An employer is only required to provide work-related accommodations if you disclose your disability to the appropriate individuals.

WHEN TO DISCLOSE YOUR DISABILITY

There is no one "right" time or place to disclose your disability. Select a confidential place in which to disclose, and allow enough time for the person to ask questions. Do not dwell on the limitations of your disability. You should weigh the pros and cons of disclosure at each point of the job search, recruitment, and hiring process and make the decision to discuss your disability when it is appropriate for you. Consider the following stages:

- in a letter of application or cover letter
- before an interview
- at the interview
- in a third-party phone call or reference
- before any drug testing for illegal drugs
- after you have a job offer
- during your course of employment
- never

HOW TO DISCLOSE YOUR DISABILITY

Preparation is essential for disclosing your disability. Effective disclosure requires that you discuss your needs and provide practical suggestions for reasonable job accommodations if they are needed. One way to become comfortable discussing your disability is to find someone you trust and practice the disclosure discussion with that person. The two of you can put together a disclosure script. It should contain relevant disability information and weave in your strengths. Always keep it positive!

WHAT TO DISCLOSE ABOUT YOUR DISABILITY

There is no required information to share about your disability. In fact, it will be different for everyone. For example, if you have an apparent disability, it is often beneficial to address how you plan to accomplish tasks required by the job. This can affirm to the employer that you are suited for the position. Additionally, by demonstrating your own ease and comfort with the job requirements, you can relay to employers other traits that are desirable in an applicant. A person with a hidden disability, on the other hand, will first need to decide whether to disclose the disability, and subsequently determine what

information to share about the disability. Generally, if you choose to disclose, it is most helpful to share the following:
- general information about your disability
- why you are disclosing your disability
- how your disability affects your ability to perform key job tasks
- types of accommodations that have worked for you in the past
- types of accommodations you anticipate needing in the workplace

TO WHOM TO DISCLOSE YOUR DISABILITY

Disclose your disability on a "need-to-know" basis. Provide further details about your disability as it applies to your work-related accommodations to the individual who can facilitate your accommodation request. Consider disclosing to the supervisor responsible for the hiring, promoting, and/or firing of employees. This person needs to be informed of your disability-related needs to provide the necessary support and judge your job performance fairly.

DISCLOSURE PROTECTIONS AND RESPONSIBILITIES

As a person with a disability, you have disclosure protections and significant responsibilities to yourself and your employers.

You are entitled to:
- have information about your disability treated confidentially and respectfully
- seek information about hiring practices from any organization
- choose to disclose your disability at any time during the employment process
- receive reasonable accommodations for an interview
- be considered for a position based on your skill and merit
- have respectful questioning about your disability for the purpose of determining whether you need accommodaions and if so, what kind

You have the responsibility to:
- disclose your need for any work-related reasonable accommodations
- bring your skills and merits to the table
- be truthful, self-determined, and proactive[1]

---

[1] "Youth, Disclosure, and the Workplace Why, When, What, and How," U.S. Department of Labor (DOL), June 6, 2007. Available online. URL: www.dol.gov/agencies/odep/publications/fact-sheets/youth-disclosure-and-the-workplace-why-when-what-and-how. Accessed August 7, 2024.

Chapter 13 | Inclusive Growth: The Role of People with Disabilities in Modern Business

By fostering a culture of diversity—a capacity to appreciate and value individual differences—in all aspects of their operations, employers benefit from varied perspectives on how to confront business challenges and achieve success.

Although the term is most often used to refer to differences among individuals such as ethnicity, gender, age, and religion, diversity actually encompasses the infinite range of individuals' unique attributes and experiences. As the nation's largest minority—comprising almost 50 million individuals—people with disabilities contribute to diversity, and businesses can enhance their competitive edge by taking steps to ensure they are integrated into their workforce and customer base.

IN THE WORKFORCE

Perhaps more than any other group, individuals with disabilities have the ability to adapt to different situations and circumstances. As employees, they add to the range of viewpoints businesses need to succeed, offering fresh ideas on how to solve problems, accomplish tasks, and implement strategies. Hiring people with disabilities can positively influence a business's bottom line. Recruiting and retaining workers with disabilities is one strategy to counter the effects of an aging and shrinking workforce. This untapped labor pool can offer a source of skilled employees and contribute to

increasing retention and reducing turnover. In addition, tax incentives and technical assistance can help with accommodations, which are often relatively easy and inexpensive to implement. To gain these benefits and others, employers should take steps to attract and retain employees with disabilities, such as:
- seeking out qualified candidates with disabilities for job openings
- establishing a system for educating all workers about the value people with disabilities bring to an organization
- incorporating a disability focus into any diversity training program
- ensuring that internal professional development programs are available to people with disabilities
- providing employees with disabilities with candid and prompt feedback on their performance in the same manner as provided for individuals without disabilities
- making certain that training and other off-site activities are accessible to employees with disabilities
- taking advantage of tax credits and educational resources to provide accommodations for both new employees with disabilities and employees returning to work following an illness or injury

IN THE MARKETPLACE

A business's commitment to diversity is also reflected in its customer base, and companies are beginning to recognize the value of people with disabilities as a target market. Organizations such as the National Organization on Disability (NOD) estimate that Americans with disabilities represent more than $200 billion in discretionary spending—not including their extended families and support networks, who are also a significant market segment. When deciding how to spend this money, individuals with disabilities have the same standards as all customers—they want quality products and services at competitive prices. To tap this market, businesses should take steps to ensure their marketing efforts convey that people with disabilities

are valued as customers and that their products and services are designed to meet their diverse needs, offering accessibility and inclusivity at every level. Such steps may include:
- incorporating people with disabilities into the business's marketing strategy
- testing proposed marketing tactics among people with disabilities
- implementing promotional tactics specifically targeted to people with disabilities
- ensuring that communication channels for advertising and promotion reach people with disabilities
- incorporating people with disabilities in advertising and other promotional activities
- recognizing that the disability market is diverse and that one size does not fit all
- defining how and why the disability market needs the business's products and services
- including people with disabilities in product development, keeping in mind that products created to meet the needs of people with disabilities often turn out to have widespread applicability
- devising simple modifications to make existing products and services accessible to people with disabilities

Incorporating people with disabilities into both the workforce and the marketplace not only enhances diversity but also drives business success. By recognizing the unique contributions of individuals with disabilities, businesses can tap into a wealth of talent and creativity, improve retention, and expand their customer base. Whether through hiring practices, professional development, or targeted marketing strategies, businesses that prioritize inclusion stand to benefit from the diverse perspectives and opportunities that people with disabilities bring to the table.[1]

---

[1] "Diverse Perspectives: People with Disabilities Fulfilling Your Business Goals," U.S. Department of Labor (DOL), October 22, 2005. Available online. URL: www.dol.gov/agencies/odep/publications/fact-sheets/diverse-perspectives-people-with-disabilities-fulfilling-your-business-goals. Accessed August 10, 2024.

Part 3 | Recovery, Rehabilitation, and Caregiving

Chapter 14 | The Importance of Early Intervention

Chapter Contents
Section 14.1—Act Early: The Power of Early Intervention................... 94
Section 14.2—Early Intervention in Childhood Hearing Loss................ 96
Section 14.3—Early Hearing Detection................................. 98

Section 14.1 | Act Early: The Power of Early Intervention

ACT EARLY ON DEVELOPMENTAL CONCERNS

Acting early on developmental concerns can make a real difference for your child and you. If you are concerned about your child's development, do not wait. You know your child best.

Early intervention helps children improve their abilities and learn new skills. Take these steps to help your child today:
- If you notice any signs of possible developmental delay, tell your child's doctor or nurse and ask for a developmental screening.
- If you or the doctor still feel worried:
  - Ask for a referral to a specialist.
  - Call your state or territory's early intervention program to determine if your child can get services to help.

WHAT IS EARLY INTERVENTION?

Early intervention:
- is the term used to describe services and support that help babies and toddlers (from birth to age three in most states/territories) with developmental delays or disabilities and their families
- may include speech therapy, physical therapy, and other types of services based on the needs of the child and family
- can significantly affect a child's ability to learn new skills and increase their success in school and life

Early intervention programs are available in every state and territory. These services are provided for free or at a reduced cost for any child who meets the state's criteria for developmental delay.

WHY IS EARLY INTERVENTION IMPORTANT?
Earlier Is Better

Intervention is likely to be more effective when it is provided earlier in life rather than later.

The connections in a baby's brain are most adaptable in the first three years of life. These connections, also called "neural circuits," are the foundation for learning, behavior, and health. Over time, these connections become harder to change.

Intervention Works

Early intervention services can change a child's developmental path and improve outcomes for children, families, and communities.

Help Your Child, Help Your Family!

Families benefit from early intervention by being better able to meet their children's needs from an early age and throughout their lives.

WHAT TO DO WHILE YOU WAIT FOR AN APPOINTMENT

Families may have to wait many weeks or months for an appointment to see a specialist or start intervention services for their child. If this happens, there are some simple things you can do to help your child's development while you wait.

- **Make the most of playtime.** Try some simple tips and activities safely, such as reading books, singing songs, and playing outside together. Talk with your child's doctor and teachers if you have questions or for more ideas on how to help your child's development.
- **Download the Centers for Disease Control and Prevention's (CDC) Milestone Tracker App.** Use the CDC's app (www.cdc.gov/milestonetracker) with illustrated checklists to track your child's development from two months to five years. The app can help you communicate with your child's doctor or early intervention contact about your child's milestones and any concerns. The app also provides tips for encouraging your child's development.[1]

---

[1] National Center on Birth Defects and Developmental Disabilities (NCBDDD), "Why Act Early If You're Concerned about Development?" Centers for Disease Control and Prevention (CDC), April 3, 2024. Available online. URL: www.cdc.gov/ncbddd/actearly/whyActEarly.html. Accessed August 9, 2024.

HOW DO YOU FIND OUT IF YOUR CHILD IS ELIGIBLE FOR SERVICES?

Eligibility for early intervention services is based on an evaluation of your child's skills and abilities.

If you, your child's doctor, or other care provider is concerned about your child's development, ask to be connected with your state or territory's early intervention program to find out if your child can get services to help. If your doctor is not able to connect you, you can reach out yourself. A doctor's referral is not necessary.

- If your child is under age three:
  - Call your state or territory's early intervention program. You can find each program's contact information at www.cdc.gov/ncbddd/actearly/parents/states.html. When you call, say, "I have concerns about my child's development and I would like to have my child evaluated to find out if he or she is eligible for early intervention services."
- If your child is three or older:
  - Call any local public elementary school (even if your child does not go there) and say, "I have concerns about my child's development, and I would like to have my child evaluated through the school system for preschool special education services."
  - If the person who answers is unfamiliar with preschool special education, ask to speak with the school or district's special education director.[2]

Section 14.2 | Early Intervention in Childhood Hearing Loss

Every state has an Early Hearing Detection and Intervention (EHDI) program, which aims to identify infants and children with hearing

---

[2] National Center on Birth Defects and Developmental Disabilities (NCBDDD), "What Is 'Early Intervention'?" Centers for Disease Control and Prevention (CDC), June 6, 2023. Available online. URL: www.cdc.gov/ncbddd/actearly/parents/states.html. Accessed August 9, 2024.

loss. The EHDI promotes timely follow-up testing and provides intervention services for families whose children are diagnosed with hearing loss.

If your child has a hearing loss or if you have any concerns about your child's hearing, call toll-free 800-CDC-INFO or contact your local EHDI program coordinator to find available services in your state.

EARLY INTERVENTION (0–3 YEARS)

Hearing loss can affect a child's ability to develop speech, language, and social skills. The earlier a child who is deaf or hard of hearing starts receiving services, the more likely the child's communication (speech or sign language) and social skills will reach their full potential.

Early intervention program services help young children with hearing loss learn communication and other important skills. Research shows that early intervention services can greatly improve a child's development.

Babies diagnosed with hearing loss should begin receiving intervention services as soon as possible, but no later than six months of age.

Many services are available through the Individuals with Disabilities Education Improvement Act 2004 (IDEA 2004). Services for children from birth through 36 months of age are Early Intervention or Part C services. Even if your child has not been diagnosed with hearing loss, they may be eligible for early intervention treatment services. IDEA 2004 states that children under the age of 3 (36 months) who are at risk of having developmental delays may be eligible for services. These services are provided through an early intervention system in your state. Through this system, you can request an evaluation.

SPECIAL EDUCATION (3–22 YEARS)

Special education is instruction specifically designed to address the educational and related developmental needs of older children with disabilities or those experiencing developmental delays. Services for these children are provided through the public school system and are available through the Individuals with IDEA 2004, Part B.

LEARNING LANGUAGE

Without extra help, children with hearing loss can struggle with language learning and may be at risk for other developmental delays.

Families with children who have hearing loss often need to change their communication habits or learn special skills (such as sign language) to help their children learn language. These skills can be used alongside hearing aids, cochlear or auditory brainstem implants, and other devices that help children hear.

FAMILY SUPPORT SERVICES

For many parents, their child's hearing loss is unexpected. Parents often need both time and support to adapt to their child's hearing loss.

Parents of children with recently identified hearing loss can seek various types of support. Support is anything that helps a family and may include advice, information, opportunities to meet other parents of children with hearing loss, finding a mentor with deafness, locating childcare or transportation, allowing parents time for personal relaxation, or simply having a supportive listener.[1]

Section 14.3 | Early Hearing Detection

HEARING SCREENING AND TESTING FOR CHILDREN

Hearing screening is a test used to determine if people might have hearing loss. Hearing screening is easy and painless, usually taking only a few minutes. If a baby or child does not pass a hearing screening, it is crucial to get a full hearing test as soon as possible. This test, also known as an "audiology evaluation," is recommended as part of the Early Hearing Detection and Intervention (EHDI) benchmarks, which include screening for hearing loss before one month of age, diagnostic evaluation before three months of age, and enrollment in early intervention before six months of age—known as the "1–3–6 benchmarks."

---

[1] "Treatment and Intervention for Hearing Loss," Centers for Disease Control and Prevention (CDC), May 15, 2024. Available online. URL: www.cdc.gov/hearing-loss-children/treatment. Accessed August 9, 2024.

WHY SHOULD A CHILD BE SCREENED OR TESTED FOR HEARING LOSS?

Hearing loss can affect a child's ability to develop communication, language, and social skills. The earlier children with hearing loss start receiving services, the more likely they are to reach their full potential. If you are a parent or caregiver and suspect your child has hearing loss, trust your instincts and speak with your doctor.

WHEN SHOULD A CHILD BE SCREENED OR TESTED FOR HEARING LOSS?
Babies
- All babies should be screened for hearing loss no later than one month of age. It is best if they are screened before leaving the hospital after birth.
- If a baby does not pass a hearing screening, it is vital to get a full hearing test as soon as possible, but no later than three months of age.

Older Babies and Children
- If you think a child might have hearing loss, ask the doctor for a hearing test as soon as possible.
- Children at risk for acquired, progressive, or delayed-onset hearing loss should have at least one hearing test by 2–2 1/2 years of age. Hearing loss that worsens over time is known as "progressive hearing loss." Hearing loss that develops after birth is called "delayed-onset" or "acquired hearing loss."
- If a child does not pass a hearing screening, it is important to get a full hearing test as soon as possible.

TYPES OF TESTS

All children who do not pass a hearing screening should have a full hearing test, also called an "audiology evaluation." An audiologist, an expert trained to test hearing, will perform the full hearing test. The audiologist will also ask questions about birth history, ear infections, and family history of hearing loss.

There are many kinds of tests an audiologist can use to determine if a person has hearing loss, how severe it is, and what type of hearing loss it is. These hearing tests are easy and painless.

Auditory Brainstem Response Test or Brainstem Auditory Evoked Response Test

- Auditory brainstem response (ABR) or brainstem auditory evoked response (BAER) is a test that checks the brain's response to sound. Because this test does not rely on a person's behavioral response, the person being tested can be sound asleep during the test.
- Auditory brainstem response focuses only on the function of the inner ear, the acoustic (hearing) nerve, and part of the brain pathways associated with hearing. For this test, electrodes are placed on the person's head (similar to electrodes placed around the heart when an electrocardiogram (ECG or EKG) is done), and brain wave activity in response to sound is recorded.

Otoacoustic Emissions

- Otoacoustic emissions (OAE) is a test that checks the inner ear's response to sound. Like the ABR test, this test does not rely on a person's behavioral response, so the person being tested can be sound asleep during the test.

Behavioral Audiometry Evaluation

- Behavioral audiometry evaluation tests how a person responds to sound overall and assesses the function of all parts of the ear. The person being tested must be awake and actively respond to sounds heard during the test.
- Infants and toddlers are observed for changes in behavior, such as sucking a pacifier, quieting, or searching for the sound. They are rewarded for the correct response by watching an animated toy (this is called "Visual Reinforcement Audiometry"). Sometimes older children are given a more play-like activity (this is called "Conditioned Play Audiometry").

The Importance of Early Intervention | 101

With the parents' permission, the audiologist will share the results with the child's primary care doctor and other specialists, such as:
- an ear, nose, and throat doctor (otolaryngologist)
- an eye doctor (ophthalmologist)
- a professional trained in genetics (clinical geneticist or genetics counselor)[1]

---

[1] "Screening for Hearing Loss," Centers for Disease Control and Prevention (CDC), May 15, 2024. Available online. URL: www.cdc.gov/hearing-loss-children/screening. Accessed August 9, 2024.

Chapter 15 | **Communication Strategies and Technologies**

Chapter Contents
Section 15.1—Communication Techniques for Individuals with Hearing Loss....104
Section 15.2—Developing Communication Skills in Children with Hearing Loss...107
Section 15.3—American Sign Language 109
Section 15.4—Assistive Devices for Enhanced Communication.............111
Section 15.5—Hearing Aids 114
Section 15.6—Cochlear Implants.....................................116

Section 15.1 | Communication Techniques for Individuals with Hearing Loss

People with hearing loss and their families often need to develop special communication skills. These skills can be used in conjunction with hearing aids, cochlear implants, and other devices that enhance hearing abilities.

AMERICAN SIGN LANGUAGE

American Sign Language (ASL) is a language itself. While English and Spanish are spoken languages, ASL is a visual language.

ASL is a complete language. People communicate using hand shapes, direction and motion of the hands, body language, and facial expressions. ASL has its own grammar, word order, and sentence structure. People can share feelings, jokes, and complete ideas using ASL.

Like any other language, ASL must be learned. People can take ASL classes and start teaching their baby even while they are still learning it. A baby can learn ASL as a first language. Also, experts in ASL can work with families to help them learn ASL.

Children can use many other skills with ASL. Finger spelling is one skill that is almost always used with ASL. Finger spelling is used to spell out words that do not have a sign—such as names of people and places.

CONCEPTUALLY ACCURATE SIGNED ENGLISH

Conceptually Accurate Signed English (CASE), sometimes called "Pidgin Signed English" (PSE), has developed between people who use ASL and people who use Manually Coded English (MCE), using signs based on ASL and MCE. This helps them understand each other better. CASE is flexible and can be changed depending on the people using it.

Other communication tools can be used with CASE. Finger spelling, for example, is often used in combination with CASE to spell out words that do not have a sign, such as names of people and places.

CUED SPEECH

Cued speech helps people who are deaf or hard of hearing better understand spoken languages.

When watching a person's mouth, many speech sounds look the same on the face even though the sounds heard are different. For instance, the words "mat," "bat," and "pat" look the same on the face even though they sound very different. When "cueing" English, the person communicating uses eight hand shapes and four places near the mouth to help the person looking tell the difference between speech sounds. Cued speech allows the person to make out sounds and words when they are using other building blocks, such as speechreading (lipreading) or auditory training (listening).

FINGER SPELLING

With finger spelling, the person uses hands and fingers to spell out words. Hand shapes represent the letters in the alphabet. Finger Spelling is used with many other communication methods; it is almost never used by itself. It is most often used with ASL, CASE, and MCE to spell out words that do not have a sign, such as the names of places or people.

LISTENING/AUDITORY TRAINING

Most people who are deaf or hard of hearing have some hearing, called "residual hearing." Some people rely on or learn how to maximize their residual hearing (auditory training). This building block is often combined with other building blocks (such as hearing aids, cochlear implants, or other assistive devices).

Listening might seem easy to a person with hearing, but for a person with hearing loss, listening is often hard without proper training. Like all other tools, the skill of listening must be learned. Often, a speech-language pathologist (SLP; a professional trained to teach people how to use speech and language) will work with the person with hearing loss and the family.

MANUALLY CODED ENGLISH

Manually Coded English comprises signs that are a visual code for spoken English. MCE is a code for a language—the English language. Many of the signs (hand shapes and hand motions) in MCE are borrowed from ASL. But unlike ASL, the grammar, word order, and sentence structure of MCE are similar to the English language.

Children and adults can use many other communication tools in addition to MCE. One that is commonly used is finger spelling, which is used to spell out words that do not have a sign in MCE, such as names of people and places.

NATURAL GESTURES

Natural gestures—or body language—are actions that people normally do to help others understand a message. For example, if a parent wants to ask a toddler if they want to be picked up, they might stretch out their arms and ask, "Up?" For an older child, the parent might motion with their arms as they call the child to come inside. Or, the parent might put a first finger over their mouth and nose to show that the child needs to be quiet.

Babies will begin to use this building block naturally if they can see what others are doing. It is not taught; it just comes naturally. It is always used with other building blocks.

SPOKEN SPEECH

People can use speech to express themselves. Speech is a skill that many people take for granted. Learning to speak is a skill that can help build language.

Speech or learning to speak is often used in combination with hearing aids, cochlear implants, or other assistive devices that help people maximize their residual hearing. A person with some residual hearing may find it easier to learn speech than a person with no residual hearing. Since speech can only be used by a person to express themselves, other building blocks—such as hearing with a hearing aid—must be added to help the person understand what is being said, so they can communicate with others.

Speaking may seem easy to a person with hearing, but for a person with hearing loss, speaking is often hard without proper training. Like all other communication tools, the skill of speaking must be learned. Often, a SLP will work with the person with hearing loss and the family.

SPEECHREADING

Speechreading (or lipreading) helps a person with hearing loss understand speech. The person watches the movements of a speaker's mouth and face and understands what the speaker is saying. About

40 percent of the sounds in the English language can be seen on the lips of a speaker in good conditions, such as a well-lit room where the child can see the speaker's face. But some words cannot be read. For example: "bop," "mop," and "pop" look exactly alike when spoken. (You can see this for yourself in a mirror.)

Children often use speechreading in combination with other tools, such as auditory training (listening), cued speech, and others. But it cannot be successful alone. Babies will naturally begin using this building block if they can see the speaker's mouth and face. But as a child gets older, he or she will still need some training.

Sometimes, when talking with a person who is deaf or hard of hearing, people will exaggerate their mouth movements or talk very loudly. Exaggerated mouth movements and a loud voice can make speechreading very hard. It is important to talk in a normal way and look directly at your child's face and make sure he or she is watching you.[1]

Section 15.2 | Developing Communication Skills in Children with Hearing Loss

It is never too early to start helping your baby learn to communicate. Without extra support, children with hearing loss may face challenges in communication, which can lead to other developmental delays. Families of children with hearing loss often need to acquire special skills to assist their children in learning to communicate. These skills can be used alongside cochlear implants and other devices that help children hear. Many parents seek guidance in learning to use these special skills. Several programs are available, each emphasizing different communication skills. Here are five programs and the skills often included in each:

AUDITORY-ORAL PROGRAM

The auditory-oral program teaches babies and young children who are deaf or hard of hearing to use whatever hearing they have.

---

[1] "How People with Hearing Loss Learn to Communicate," Centers for Disease Control and Prevention (CDC), May 15, 2024. Available online. URL: www.cdc.gov/hearing-loss-children/treatment/how-people-with-hearing-loss-learn-language.html. Accessed August 10, 2024.

They also use lipreading (speechreading) and gestures to understand and use spoken language. This program includes building blocks such as natural gestures, listening, speech (lip) reading, and speech.

AUDITORY-VERBAL PROGRAM

The auditory-verbal program teaches babies and young children who are deaf or hard of hearing to use their amplified residual hearing or hearing through electrical stimulation (cochlear implants) to listen, understand spoken language, and speak. This program includes building blocks such as listening and speech.

BILINGUAL PROGRAM

This program teaches babies and young children who are deaf or hard of hearing two languages—American Sign Language (ASL) and the family's native language (e.g., English or Spanish). ASL is usually taught as the child's first language, and English (or the family's native language) is taught as the child's second language through reading, writing, speech, and the use of residual hearing. This program also promotes respect for Deaf and hearing cultures and includes building blocks such as finger spelling and natural gestures.

CUED SPEECH (BUILDING BLOCK) PROGRAM

Cued speech (sometimes called "cueing") is a building block that helps children who are deaf or hard of hearing better understand spoken languages. Many speech sounds look the same on the face, even though the sounds are different. For instance, the words "mat," "bat," and "pat" look the same on the lips and mouth. When "cueing" English, the person communicating uses eight hand shapes and four locations near the mouth to help distinguish between speechsounds.

TOTAL COMMUNICATION PROGRAM

This program teaches babies and young children who are deaf or hard of hearing to use a combination of building blocks to communicate in the English language. Most Total Communication programs use some form of simultaneous communication (speaking and signing at the same time). This program includes building blocks such as Conceptually Accurate Signed English (CASE), finger spelling, listening, Manually Coded English (MCE), natural gestures, speech (lip) reading, and speech.

As a parent, you can review these programs and select the skill—or set of skills—that will best help your child communicate. Some parents choose a single program because it works best for their child, while others select skills from two or more programs to achieve the best results. You can also consult with your team of health-care professionals to determine which program(s) will give your child the greatest chance for success.[1]

Section 15.3 | American Sign Language

WHAT IS AMERICAN SIGN LANGUAGE?
American Sign Language (ASL) is a complete, natural language with linguistic properties similar to spoken languages, though its grammar differs from English. ASL is expressed through movements of the hands and face. It serves as the primary language for many North Americans who are deaf or hard of hearing and is also used by some hearing people.

IS SIGN LANGUAGE THE SAME IN OTHER COUNTRIES?
There is no universal sign language. Different sign languages are used in various countries or regions. For example, British Sign Language (BSL) is distinct from ASL, meaning that Americans familiar with ASL may not understand BSL. Some countries incorporate features of ASL into their sign languages.

WHERE DID AMERICAN SIGN LANGUAGE ORIGINATE?
No single person or committee invented ASL. The exact origins of ASL are unclear, but some suggest it arose more than 200 years ago from the intermixing of local sign languages and French Sign

---

[1] "Building Communication Skills," Centers for Disease Control and Prevention (CDC), May 15, 2024. Available online. URL: www.cdc.gov/hearing-loss-children-guide/parents-guide/building-languages.html. Accessed August 10, 2024.

Language (Langue des Signes Française, or LSF). Today's ASL includes elements of LSF and the original local sign languages, which have evolved into a rich, complex, and mature language. Modern ASL and LSF are now distinct languages; while they still share some signs, they are no longer mutually intelligible.

HOW DOES AMERICAN SIGN LANGUAGE COMPARE WITH SPOKEN LANGUAGE?

American Sign Language is entirely separate and distinct from English. It has all the fundamental features of language, including its own rules for pronunciation, word formation, and word order. While every language has methods of signaling different functions, such as asking a question instead of making a statement, these methods differ across languages. For example, English speakers might ask a question by raising the pitch of their voices and adjusting word order, whereas ASL users ask a question by raising their eyebrows, widening their eyes, and tilting their bodies forward.

As with other languages, the ways of expressing ideas in ASL vary among its users. In addition to individual differences in expression, ASL features regional accents and dialects. Just as certain English words are pronounced differently in various parts of the country, ASL exhibits regional variations in signing rhythm, pronunciation, slang, and the signs used. Other sociological factors, including age and gender, also influence ASL usage and contribute to its variety, similar to spoken languages.

Finger spelling is an integral part of ASL and is used to spell out English words. In the finger-spelled alphabet, each letter corresponds to a distinct handshape. Finger spelling is often employed for proper names or to indicate the English word for something.

HOW DO MOST CHILDREN LEARN AMERICAN SIGN LANGUAGE?

Parents are typically the primary source of a child's early language acquisition, but for children who are deaf, additional people may serve as language models. A child with deafness born to parents who already use ASL will naturally acquire ASL, just as a hearing child learns spoken language from hearing parents. However, for a child with deafness and hearing parents who have no prior experience with ASL, language acquisition may differ. In fact, 9 out of 10 children born with deafness have hearing parents. Some hearing parents choose to introduce sign language to their children, learning it alongside them. Children with deafness and hearing parents often learn sign language through their deaf peers and become fluent over time.

WHY EMPHASIZE EARLY LANGUAGE LEARNING?

It is essential for parents to expose a child with deafness or hearing loss to language (spoken or signed) as early as possible. The sooner a child is exposed to and begins to acquire language, the better their language, cognitive, and social development will be. Research indicates that the first few years of life are critical for language skill development, with even the early months of life being vital for establishing effective communication with caregivers. Due to screening programs in place at almost all hospitals in the United States and its territories, newborns are tested for hearing before they leave the hospital. If a baby has hearing loss, this screening allows parents to learn about communication options and start their child's language learning process during this crucial early stage of development.[1]

Section 15.4 | Assistive Devices for Enhanced Communication

WHAT ARE ASSISTIVE DEVICES?

The terms "assistive device" or "assistive technology" can refer to any device that helps a person with hearing loss or a voice, speech, or language disorder to communicate. These terms often describe devices that help a person hear and understand what is being said

---

[1] "American Sign Language," National Institute on Deafness and Other Communication Disorders (NIDCD), October 29, 2021. Available online. URL: www.nidcd.nih.gov/health/american-sign-language. Accessed August 10, 2024.

more clearly or express thoughts more easily. With the development of digital and wireless technologies, an increasing number of devices are becoming available to help people with hearing, voice, speech, and language disorders communicate more effectively and participate more fully in their daily lives.

WHAT TYPES OF ASSISTIVE DEVICES ARE AVAILABLE?

Health professionals use various names to describe assistive devices:
- Assistive listening devices (ALDs) help amplify the sounds you want to hear, especially in environments with significant background noise. ALDs can be used with a hearing aid or cochlear implant to help the wearer hear specific sounds more clearly.
- Augmentative and alternative communication (AAC) devices assist people with communication disorders in expressing themselves. These devices range from a simple picture board to a computer program synthesizing speech from text.
- Alerting devices connect to a doorbell, telephone, or alarm that emits a loud sound or blinking light to notify someone with hearing loss that an event is occurring.

WHAT TYPES OF ASSISTIVE LISTENING DEVICES ARE AVAILABLE?

Several types of ALDs are available to improve sound transmission for people with hearing loss. Some are designed for large facilities such as classrooms, theaters, places of worship, and airports. Other types are intended for personal use in small settings and one-on-one conversations. All can be used with or without hearing aids or a cochlear implant. ALD systems for large facilities include hearing loop systems, frequency-modulated (FM) systems, and infrared systems.

WHAT TYPES OF AUGMENTATIVE AND ALTERNATIVE COMMUNICATION DEVICES ARE AVAILABLE FOR FACE-TO-FACE COMMUNICATION?

The simplest AAC device is a picture board or touch screen that uses pictures or symbols of typical items and activities in a person's daily life. For example, a person might touch the image of a glass to ask for a drink. Many picture boards can be customized and expanded based on a person's age, education, occupation, and interests.

Keyboards, touch screens, and sometimes a person's limited speech may be used to communicate desired words. Some devices employ a text display. The display panel typically faces outward so that two people can exchange information while facing each other. Spelling and word prediction software can make it faster and easier to enter information.

Speech-generating devices go one step further by translating words or pictures into speech. Some models allow users to choose from several different voices, such as male or female, child or adult, and even some regional accents. Some devices employ a vocabulary of prerecorded words, while others have an unlimited vocabulary, synthesizing speech as words are typed in. Software programs that convert personal computers into speaking devices are also available.

WHAT TYPES OF ALERTING DEVICES ARE AVAILABLE?

Alerting or alarm devices use sound, light, vibrations, or a combination of these techniques to notify someone when a particular event occurs. Clocks and wake-up alarm systems allow a person to choose to wake up to flashing lights, horns, or gentle shaking.

Visual alert signalers monitor various household devices and other sounds, such as doorbells and telephones. When the phone rings, the visual alert signaler is activated and will vibrate or flash a light to notify people. In addition, remote receivers placed around the house can alert a person from any room. Portable vibrating pagers can notify parents and caretakers when a baby is crying. Some baby monitoring devices analyze a baby's cry and light up a picture to indicate if the baby sounds hungry, bored, or sleepy.[1]

---

[1] "Assistive Devices for People with Hearing, Voice, Speech, or Language Disorders," National Institute on Deafness and Other Communication Disorders (NIDCD), November 12, 2019. Available online. URL: www.nidcd.nih.gov/health/assistive-devices-people-hearing-voice-speech-or-language-disorders. Accessed August 10, 2024.

Section 15.5 | Hearing Aids

WHAT IS A HEARING AID?

A hearing aid is a small electronic device worn in or behind the ear. It amplifies certain sounds, enabling a person with hearing loss to listen, communicate, and participate more fully in daily activities. Hearing aids can enhance hearing in both quiet and noisy environments, yet only about one in five people who could benefit from one actually uses one.

A hearing aid consists of three basic components:
- a microphone
- an amplifier
- a speaker

The microphone picks up sound, converting sound waves into electrical signals, which are then sent to the amplifier. The amplifier increases the strength of these signals and sends them to the ear via the speaker.

HOW CAN HEARING AIDS HELP?

Hearing aids are particularly useful for improving hearing and speech comprehension in individuals with sensorineural hearing loss, a condition caused by damage to the small sensory cells in the inner ear, known as "hair cells." This type of hearing loss may result from disease, aging, noise exposure, or certain medications.

Hearing aids magnify sound vibrations entering the ear. Surviving hair cells detect these amplified vibrations and convert them into neural signals, which are then transmitted to the brain. The severity of hearing loss determines the amount of amplification needed. However, there are practical limits to the amplification a hearing aid can provide. If the inner ear is severely damaged, even large vibrations may not be converted into neural signals, rendering a hearing aid ineffective.

WHERE CAN I GET HELP WITH MY HEARING LOSS?

If you or a family member has concerns about hearing loss, several options are available. Over-the-counter (OTC) hearing aids are a new category of hearing aids that can be purchased directly without

Communication Strategies and Technologies | 115

consulting a hearing health professional. These aids are designed for adults with perceived mild to moderate hearing loss. For more significant or complicated hearing loss, prescription hearing aids are available from a hearing health professional, who will program them according to your specific needs.

WHAT QUESTIONS SHOULD I ASK BEFORE BUYING A HEARING AID?

Before purchasing a hearing aid, consider asking your audiologist the following questions:
- What features would be most beneficial for my hearing needs?
- What is the total cost of the hearing aid? Do the advantages of newer technologies justify the higher cost?
- Is there a trial period to test the hearing aids? (Most manufacturers offer a 30- to 60-day trial period during which aids can be returned for a refund.) What fees are nonrefundable if the aids are returned after the trial period?
- How long is the warranty? Can it be extended? Does it cover future maintenance and repairs?
- Can the audiologist make adjustments, provide servicing, and handle minor repairs? Will loaner aids be available when repairs are needed?
- What instruction and support does the audiologist offer?

HOW CAN I CARE FOR MY HEARING AID?

Proper maintenance and care are essential for extending the life of your hearing aid. Consider the following tips:
- Keep hearing aids away from heat and moisture.
- Clean hearing aids as instructed; earwax and ear drainage can damage them.
- Avoid using hairspray or other hair care products while wearing hearing aids.
- Turn off hearing aids when not in use.
- Replace dead batteries promptly.
- Keep replacement batteries and small hearing aids out of reach of children and pets.

CAN I OBTAIN FINANCIAL ASSISTANCE FOR A HEARING AID?

Hearing aids are generally not covered by health insurance, though some exceptions exist. For eligible children and young adults up to age 21, Medicaid covers the diagnosis and treatment of hearing loss, including hearing aids, under the Early and Periodic Screening, Diagnostic, and Treatment (EPSDT) service. Additionally, children may receive coverage through their state's early intervention program or State Children's Health Insurance Program (SCHIP).[1]

Section 15.6 | Cochlear Implants

WHAT IS A COCHLEAR IMPLANT?

A cochlear implant is a small, complex electronic device that can provide a sense of sound to individuals who are profoundly deaf or severely hard of hearing. The implant consists of two main parts: an external portion that sits behind the ear and an internal portion that is surgically placed under the skin. The components of a cochlear implant include:

- **Microphone.** Picks up sound from the environment.
- **Speech processor.** Selects and arranges sounds picked up by the microphone.
- **Transmitter and receiver/stimulator.** Receive signals from the speech processor and convert them into electric impulses.
- **Electrode array.** A group of electrodes that collects the impulses from the stimulator and sends them to different regions of the auditory nerve.

A cochlear implant does not restore normal hearing. Instead, it provides a person with deafness a useful representation of sounds in the environment and helps them understand speech.

---

[1] "Hearing Aids," National Institute on Deafness and Other Communication Disorders (NIDCD), October 11, 2022. Available online. URL: www.nidcd.nih.gov/health/hearing-aids. Accessed August 10, 2024.

HOW DOES A COCHLEAR IMPLANT WORK?
A cochlear implant differs significantly from a hearing aid. While hearing aids amplify sounds to be detected by damaged ears, cochlear implants bypass the damaged portions of the ear and directly stimulate the auditory nerve. The signals generated by the implant are sent via the auditory nerve to the brain, which recognizes them as sound. Hearing through a cochlear implant differs from normal hearing and requires time to learn or relearn. However, it allows many individuals to recognize warning signals, understand environmental sounds, and comprehend speech in person or over the telephone.

HOW DOES SOMEONE RECEIVE A COCHLEAR IMPLANT?
Receiving a cochlear implant involves both a surgical procedure and significant therapy to learn or relearn the sense of hearing. Performance with this device varies among individuals. The decision to receive an implant should involve discussions with medical specialists, including an experienced cochlear implant surgeon. The process can be costly, and while health insurance may cover the expense, this is not always the case. Some individuals may choose not to have a cochlear implant for various personal reasons. Although surgical implantations are generally safe, complications are a potential risk, as with any surgery. Additionally, learning to interpret the sounds created by an implant takes time and practice. Speech-language pathologists (SLPs) and audiologists are often involved in this learning process. All of these factors should be carefully considered before implantation.[1]

WHAT DETERMINES THE SUCCESS OF COCHLEAR IMPLANTS?
Several factors influence the success of cochlear implants, including:
- **Duration of deafness.** Patients who have been deaf for a shorter period generally experience better outcomes than those who have been deaf for a longer time.
- **Age at onset of deafness.** Success may depend on whether the patient became deaf before or after acquiring speech.

---

[1] "Cochlear Implants," National Institute on Deafness and Other Communication Disorders (NIDCD), June 13, 2024. Available online. URL: www.nidcd.nih.gov/health/cochlear-implants. Accessed August 10, 2024.

- **Age at implantation.** Younger patients, particularly those who were implanted soon after becoming deaf, tend to have better outcomes compared to older patients who have been deaf for an extended period.
- **Duration of implant use.** The length of time the patient has been using the implant can affect their success, with longer use often leading to better outcomes.
- **Learning ability.** The speed at which patients learn to use the implant plays a significant role in their success.
- **Support structure.** The quality and dedication of the patient's learning support structure, including family, educators, and therapists, are crucial for success.
- **Health and structure of the cochlea.** The condition of the cochlea, including the number of functioning nerve (spiral ganglion) cells, can affect the effectiveness of the implant.
- **Implantation variables.** Factors such as the depth of electrode insertion, the type of electrode used, and the signal processing technique can influence outcomes.
- **Patient's intelligence and communicativeness.** The cognitive abilities and communication skills of the patient also play a role in determining the success of the cochlear implant.[2]

WHAT ARE THE BENEFITS OF COCHLEAR IMPLANTS?

For people with implants, the benefits can vary:
- **Hearing ranges.** From near-normal ability to understand speech to no hearing benefit at all.
- **Adults.** Often benefit immediately, with continued improvement over approximately three months following the initial tuning sessions. Performance may continue to improve for several years.

---

[2] "What Is a Cochlear Implant?" U.S. Food and Drug Administration (FDA), February 4, 2018. Available online. URL: www.fda.gov/medical-devices/cochlear-implants/what-cochlear-implant. Accessed August 10, 2024.

Communication Strategies and Technologies | 119

- **Children**. May improve at a slower pace, requiring extensive training after implantation to help them utilize their new sense of hearing.
- **Sound perception**. Most recipients perceive loud, medium, and soft sounds and can distinguish various types of sounds, such as footsteps, door slams, engine noises, ringing phones, barking dogs, tea kettle whistles, rustling leaves, and light switches.
- **Speech understanding**. Many can understand speech without lipreading. Even when this is not possible, the implant often aids in lipreading.
- **Telephone use**. Many can make telephone calls and understand familiar voices over the phone. Some may even make regular calls and understand unfamiliar speakers, though not all implant users can use the phone effectively.
- **Television and radio**. Many can watch TV more easily, especially when they can also see the speaker's face, though listening to the radio may be more challenging without visual cues.
- **Music enjoyment**. Some recipients can enjoy music, appreciating certain instruments or voices, while others may not hear well enough to enjoy music.[3]

---

[3] "Benefits and Risks of Cochlear Implants," U.S. Food and Drug Administration (FDA), February 9, 2021. Available online. URL: www.fda.gov/medical-devices/cochlear-implants/benefits-and-risks-cochlear-implants. Accessed August 10, 2024.

Chapter 16 | **Speech-Language Pathology**

Chapter Contents
Section 16.1—Roles and Responsibilities of Speech-Language Pathologists 122
Section 16.2—Speech Therapy for Veterans 124
Section 16.3—Speech-Language Therapy for Autism Spectrum Disorder 126

Section 16.1 | Roles and Responsibilities of Speech-Language Pathologists

SPEECH-LANGUAGE PATHOLOGISTS
Speech-language pathologists (SLPs), or speech therapists, assess and treat individuals with speech, language, voice, and fluency disorders. They also assist clients with swallowing problems.

KEY RESPONSIBILITIES OF SPEECH-LANGUAGE PATHOLOGISTS
Speech-language pathologists typically perform the following duties:
- **Evaluate speech and language difficulties**. Assess levels of speech, language, or swallowing difficulty.
- **Identify client goals**. Collaborate with clients to set specific treatment goals.
- **Create and implement treatment plans**. Develop an individualized treatment plan that addresses specific functional needs.
- **Teach and train clients**. Instruct clients on how to make sounds, improve their voices, and maintain fluency.
- **Enhance communication skills**. Assist clients in enhancing vocabulary and sentence structure.
- **Swallowing therapy**. Aid clients to develop and strengthen the muscles used to swallow.
- **Counseling and support**. Offer guidance and support to clients and their families on how to cope with communication and swallowing disorders.

Speech-language pathologists work with clients who experience speech and language problems, including related cognitive or social communication challenges. Clients may have difficulty speaking, such as being unable to speak or speaking too loudly or softly. They may also have issues with rhythm and fluency, such as stuttering. SLPs also assist clients who have problems understanding language.

USE OF ALTERNATIVE COMMUNICATION SYSTEMS
Speech-language pathologists may select alternative communication systems and instruct clients in their use. They must also record their evaluations and assessments, track treatment progress, and note any changes in a client's condition or treatment plan.

SPECIALIZATION AREAS
Some SLPs specialize in working with specific age groups, such as children or older adults. Others focus on treatment programs for specific communication or swallowing problems that result from developmental delays or from medical causes, such as a stroke or a cleft palate. Still, others research topics related to speech and language issues.

COLLABORATION WITH OTHER PROFESSIONALS
Speech-language pathologists collaborate with a diverse team of health-care professionals, including:
- physicians and surgeons
- social workers
- psychologists
- occupational therapists
- physical therapists
- respiratory therapists
- audiologists
- other health-care workers

In educational settings, SLPs evaluate students for speech and language disorders and work with teachers, other school personnel, and parents to develop and carry out individual or group programs, provide counseling, and support classroom activities.[1]

---

[1] U.S. Bureau of Labor Statistics (BLS), "Speech-Language Pathologists," U.S. Department of Labor (DOL), April 17, 2024. Available online. URL: www.bls.gov/ooh/healthcare/speech-language-pathologists.htm#tab-2. Accessed August 10, 2024.

Section 16.2 | Speech Therapy for Veterans

When most people think of speech therapy or rehabilitation, they likely envision children learning to pronounce words correctly. However, in U.S. Department of Veterans Affairs (VA), speech pathologists serve individuals and service members of all ages by treating disorders that affect the entire communication system, including the brain.

Individuals who have suffered from trauma or illness may experience problems with forgetfulness, problem-solving, responding accurately, understanding jokes, following directions, or interacting with others. These issues may indicate a cognitive-communication disorder.

The good news is that, with the assistance of a speech-language pathologist (SPL), people can work to improve their cognitive skills and learn strategies to enhance their cognitive functioning, ultimately improving their quality of life (QOL).

More than 400 SPLs across the VA provide screening, evaluation, cognitive rehabilitation, and treatment for various communication and swallowing disorders.

WHY WAS I REFERRED TO SPEECH THERAPY?

This question often arises when individuals are referred to a speech pathologist. The Durham VA Speech Pathology Clinic, along with many other VA clinics, offers rehabilitation for cognitive-communication problems where trained speech pathologists provide education, training, and strategies for coping with problems following brain injury, trauma, or stroke.

Carol Smith Hammond, a speech pathologist at Durham VA, begins each patient visit by asking questions such as:
- "Do you have problems with attention or memory?"
- "Do you have issues with organization or forgetting daily tasks?"
- "Are you struggling at work or studying for college courses?"

The veterans Dr. Hammond treats were once active and successful military members. Following trauma or injury, they often experience mild cognitive problems. Many also have coexisting conditions such as anxiety, depression, posttraumatic stress disorder, or sleep disturbances, which can disrupt their ability to pay attention or concentrate.

"Patients often come to see me and are crying," said Dr. Hammond. "They are so worried about losing their job or flunking out of school."

ENHANCING LIVES WITH PRACTICAL TOOLS AND SUPPORT

During the first meeting with a veteran, Dr. Hammond immediately provides key strategies for increasing focus and concentration. She advises patients to "stop and plan" before starting the day or a new task. She also recommends simple tools such as a daily planner and a whiteboard to organize each day and check off completed tasks.

In each session, Dr. Hammond incorporates mindfulness training or meditation to help patients clear their minds of all negative thoughts or fears of failure when tackling a difficult project or preparing for a busy day. Most patients complete an average of eight speech pathology appointments, and many participate in group programs.

Recently, Dr. Hammond worked with a veteran in North Carolina who is now a farmer. He described making multiple trips between his house and the farm each day because he would forget his planned tasks and leave objects in the wrong places.

He often became frustrated and angry with family members. After cognitive rehabilitation, he commented, "The one strategy—to stop and plan each day—has changed my life."

TELEHEALTH OPTIONS WITH CONVENIENT SUPPORT

The VA speech pathology services are available for both in-person and telehealth visits. In February 2021, Durham VA provided cognitive rehabilitation using VA Video Connect technology for more than 50 veterans. VA speech pathologists completed more than 93,000 telehealth visits nationwide in 2021.

Veterans participating in cognitive rehabilitation range from 20 to 40 years old. They work, attend college courses, and many of them also have young children to care for at home. Telehealth visits provide veterans with an easy, convenient way to access VA health care when and where they need it.[1]

Section 16.3 | Speech-Language Therapy for Autism Spectrum Disorder

Speech-language therapy offers vital support for individuals with autism spectrum disorder (ASD), enhancing their ability to communicate and interact effectively with others.

VERBAL SKILLS
This therapy can significantly improve various verbal skills, including:
- **Naming.** Enhancing the ability to correctly identify and name people and objects.
- **Expressing emotions.** Improving the expression of feelings and emotions through words.
- **Language use.** Refining the use of words and construction of sentences.
- **Speech dynamics.** Enhancing the rate and rhythm of speech for clearer communication.

NONVERBAL COMMUNICATION
Beyond verbal skills, speech-language therapy also focuses on nonverbal communication, such as:
- **Sign language.** Teaching hand signals or sign language to facilitate communication.
- **Visual aids.** Using picture symbols for communication, often through systems like the Picture Exchange Communication System (PECS).

---

[1] "Why Was I Referred to Speech Therapy?" U.S. Department of Veterans Affairs (VA), May 17, 2022. Available online. URL: https://news.va.gov/103458/why-was-i-referred-to-speech-therapy. Accessed August 10, 2024.

SOCIAL INTERACTION SKILLS

Additionally, therapy sessions may include ways to improve social skills and behaviors, which are crucial for smoother interactions. For example:

- **Eye contact.** Training in maintaining appropriate eye contact during conversations.
- **Spatial awareness.** Learning to maintain a comfortable distance from others during interactions.

These elements of speech-language therapy are designed to make everyday interactions more manageable and fulfilling for individuals with ASD.[1]

---

[1] "Speech-Language Therapy for Autism," *Eunice Kennedy Shriver* National Institute of Child Health and Human Development (NICHD), April 20, 2021. Available online. URL: www.nichd.nih.gov/health/topics/autism/conditioninfo/treatments/speech-language. Accessed August 10, 2024.

Chapter 17 | **Overcoming Learning Challenges**

WHAT ARE LEARNING DISABILITIES?
Learning disabilities affect how a person learns to read, write, speak, and do math. Differences in the brain cause them, most often in how it functions and sometimes in its structure. These differences affect the way the brain processes information. Having a learning disability, or even several disabilities, is not related to intelligence. It simply means that the person's brain works differently from others. In many cases, there are interventions—treatments—that can help a person with learning disabilities read, write, speak, and calculate just as well as or better than someone without these disabilities.

Learning disabilities are often discovered once a child is in school and has learning difficulties that do not improve over time. A person can have more than one learning disability. Learning disabilities can last a person's entire life, but they can still be successful with the right educational support.

WHAT ARE SOME SIGNS OF LEARNING DISABILITIES?
Many children have trouble reading, writing, or performing other learning-related tasks at some point. This does not mean they have learning disabilities. A child with a learning disability often has several related signs, and they do not go away or get better over time. Each learning disability has its own signs, and a person with a particular disability may not have all the signs of that disability.

Children being taught in a second language may show signs of learning problems or a learning disability. The learning disability assessment must consider whether a student is bilingual or a second language learner. Additionally, for English-speaking children, the assessment should be sensitive to differences that may be due to dialect, a form of language specific to a region or group.

Common signs that a person may have learning disabilities include the following:
- problems reading and/or writing
- problems with math
- poor memory
- problems paying attention
- trouble following directions
- clumsiness
- trouble telling time
- problems staying organized

WHAT ARE THE TREATMENTS FOR LEARNING DISABILITIES?

Learning disabilities have no cure, but early intervention can lessen their effects. People with learning disabilities can develop ways to cope with their disabilities. Getting help earlier increases the chance of success in school and later in life. If learning disabilities remain untreated, a child may begin to feel frustrated, which can lead to low self-esteem and other problems.

TIPS FOR MANAGING A LEARNING DISABILITY IN ADULTHOOD

Schools can provide support to improve elementary and secondary students' math, reading, and other language skills. But how can people with learning disabilities prepare for the demands of university or working life?

- **Be your own advocate**. It is important to know and speak up for what you need. Understand your learning challenges, identify possible solutions, and ask for the resources that will allow you to reach your goals.
- **Ensure that your surroundings facilitate success**. Work with your school or employer to create a supportive learning environment, such as access to software to help you succeed now and in the future.

- **Take advantage of assistive technology.** Use computer tools customized to your own pace and needs that can read text aloud, help you articulate your thoughts, and provide structure to your writing.[1]

---

[1] "Learning Disabilities," *Eunice Kennedy Shriver* National Institute of Child Health and Human Development (NICHD), September 11, 2018. Available online. URL: www.nichd.nih.gov/health/topics/learning/conditioninfo/treatment/mld. Accessed August 10, 2024.

Chapter 18 | Tips for Caregivers of People with Disabilities

Caring for a family member with a disability, whether a child or an adult, involves balancing personal, caregiving, and everyday needs, which can be challenging. The following tips aim to help family caregivers stay safe and healthy while providing the best care possible for their loved ones.

BE INFORMED
- **Gather information**. Learn about your family member's condition and discuss their needs with other caregivers. This knowledge will enable you to make informed health decisions and better understand the challenges your family might face.
- **Observe care practices**. Notice how others care for the person with special needs and be vigilant for signs of mental or physical abuse.

GET SUPPORT
- **Seek assistance**. Family members and friends often want to help. Identify tasks they can assist with, whether big or small.
- **Join support groups**. Local or online support groups provide an opportunity to share information and connect with others facing similar experiences. These groups can combat isolation and fear, offering a network of support.

- **Utilize resources**. Friends, family, health-care providers, community services, and counselors are all available to support you and your family.

BE AN ADVOCATE
- **Advocate effectively**. As an advocate, you can better secure necessary services for your family member. Ask questions and ensure other caregivers are informed about special conditions or circumstances.
- **Document medical history**. Keep an updated medical history of your family member with a disability.
- **Communicate with employers**. Discuss your circumstances and limitations with your employer, and arrange for flexible scheduling when needed.
- **Know legal protections**. Familiarize yourself with the Americans with Disabilities Act (ADA), the Family Medical Leave Act (FMLA), and other relevant laws.

BE EMPOWERING
- **Focus on abilities**. Highlight what you and your family member with a disability can do. Celebrate milestones and, when possible, let them answer questions to empower them.
- **Promote independence**. Teach your family member to be as independent and self-assured as possible, while always considering health and safety challenges.

TAKE CARE OF YOURSELF
- **Maintain your health**. Stay healthy for yourself and those you care for. Maintain personal interests, hobbies, and friendships to avoid being consumed by caregiving.
- **Set realistic expectations**. Aim for balance and delegate tasks to others when possible. Allow yourself to take breaks, both short and long, to recharge.
- **Monitor your health**. Do not ignore signs of illness. Seek medical care when needed. Pay attention to your mental and emotional well-being. Exercise and eat healthily.

KEEP BALANCE IN THE FAMILY
- **Attend to all family members.** Ensure that you spend time with all family members, not just the one with a disability. Parents should also spend time with each other and any other children.
- **Consider respite care.** Respite care provides temporary relief, allowing families to take a break from daily caregiving routines.

EMERGENCY AND DISASTER PREPAREDNESS
It is important for people with disabilities and their caregivers to make plans to protect themselves in the event of an emergency or disaster. Emergencies and disasters can strike quickly and without warning, potentially forcing people to leave their homes or remain confined within them. For millions of Americans with disabilities, emergencies such as acts of terrorism, fires, and floods present significant challenges.

By following these tips, family caregivers can better manage their responsibilities while maintaining their own health and well-being, creating a more positive and balanced family environment.[1]

---

[1] National Center on Birth Defects and Developmental Disabilities (NCBDDD), "Disability and Health Information for Family Caregivers," Centers for Disease Control and Prevention (CDC), September 16, 2020. Available online. URL: www.cdc.gov/ncbddd/disabilityandhealth/family.html. Accessed August 10, 2024.

Chapter 19 | Speech to Speech Relay Service

Speech to Speech (STS) is a form of Telecommunications Relay Service (TRS) that allows individuals with speech disabilities to make telephone calls, either using their own voice or an assistive voice device. STS uses Communications Assistants (CAs) to relay the conversation back and forth between the person with the speech disability and the other party to the call. STS CAs are specifically trained in understanding a variety of speech disorders, which enables them to repeat what the caller says in a manner that makes the caller's words clear and understandable to the called party.

WHO USES SPEECH TO SPEECH?

Often, people with speech disabilities cannot communicate by telephone because the parties they are calling cannot understand their speech. Individuals with cerebral palsy (CP), multiple sclerosis (MS), muscular dystrophy (MD), Parkinson's disease (PD), and those who are coping with limitations from a stroke or traumatic brain injury (TBI) may have speech disabilities. People who stutter or have had a laryngectomy may also have difficulty being understood. In general, anyone with a speech disability or anyone who wishes to call someone with a speech disability can use STS.

HOW TO MAKE AND RECEIVE SPEECH TO SPEECH

A person can make an STS call from any telephone. Dial 711 to reach the relay center and indicate your wish to make an STS call. You are then connected to an STS CA who will repeat your spoken words, making them clear to the other party. Persons with speech disabilities may also receive STS calls. The calling party calls the relay center by dialing 711 and asks the CA to call the person with a speech disability. STS users have the option of muting their voices during an STS call (so that the party to whom they are speaking hears only the voice of the STS CA, and not the voice of the STS user). If you wish to use this option, please inform the STS CA to mute your voice for the other party to the call. If you choose this option, the STS CA will still be able to hear what you are saying and will re-voice what you say to the other party.

MANDATORY MINIMUM STANDARDS FOR SPEECH TO SPEECH

The Federal Communications Commission (FCC) imposes mandatory minimum standards on providers of all forms of TRS, such as ensuring user confidentiality, making service available 24 hours a day, seven days a week, and answering 85 percent of calls within 10 seconds. The FCC also imposes certain additional requirements on STS providers. For example, for each STS call lasting 20 minutes or longer, an STS CA must remain with a call for at least 20 minutes before transferring the call to another CA. This allows for more effective communication for the STS user because the same CA stays on the call for a longer time. Additionally:

- An STS CA may, at the user's request, retain information from a particular call to facilitate the completion of consecutive calls. The user may ask the TRS CA to retain such information, or the CA may ask the user if they want the CA to repeat the same information during subsequent calls. The STS CA may retain the information only for as long as it takes to complete the subsequent calls.
- STS providers must offer STS users the option to maintain a list of names and telephone numbers that the STS user commonly calls at the relay center. When the STS user requests one of these names, the CA must repeat the name and state the telephone number to the STS user. This information must be transferred to any new STS provider.
- STS providers must have emergency call procedures if an STS user calls 911.

Speech to Speech Relay Service

A list of toll-free phone numbers to access STS for each state can be obtained from this website: www.fcc.gov/general/speech-speech-services-access-numbers.[1]

---

[1] "Speech to Speech Relay Service," Federal Communications Commission (FCC), January 27, 2021. Available online. URL: www.fcc.gov/consumers/guides/speech-speech-relay-service. Accessed August 10, 2024.

Chapter 20 | Telecommunications Relay Service

Telecommunications Relay Service (TRS) allows persons with hearing or speech disabilities to place and receive telephone calls. TRS is available for local and/or long-distance calls in all 50 states, the District of Columbia, Puerto Rico, and the U.S. territories.

Telecommunications Relay Service providers are compensated for the costs of providing TRS from either a state or a federal fund. The FCC does not require an IP relay.

Telecommunications Relay Service providers must ensure user confidentiality, and Communications Assistants (with a limited exception for STS) may not keep records of any conversation's contents. Users of Voice over Internet Protocol (VoIP) service can also access relay services by dialing 711.

WHAT FORMS OF TELECOMMUNICATIONS RELAY SERVICE ARE AVAILABLE?

There are several forms of TRS, depending on the particular needs of the user and the equipment available:
- **Text-to-Voice TTY-based TRS**. This "traditional" TRS service uses a TTY to call the CA at the relay center. TTYs have a keyboard and allow people to type their telephone conversations. The text is read on a display screen and/or a paper printout. A TTY user calls a TRS relay center and types the number of the person he or she wishes to call. The CA at the relay center then makes a voice telephone call to the other party to the call, and relays the call back

and forth between the parties by speaking what a text user types, and typing what a voice telephone user speaks.
- **Voice Carry Over**. This service allows a person with a hearing disability who wants to use his or her own voice to speak directly to the called party and receive responses in text from the CA. The calling party requires no typing. This service is particularly useful for senior citizens who have lost their hearing but can still speak.
- **Hearing Carry Over**. This service allows a person with a speech disability who wants to use his or her own hearing to listen to the called party and type his or her part of the conversation on a TTY. The CA reads these words to the called party, and the caller hears responses directly from the called party.
- **Speech-to-Speech Relay Service**. Used by a person with a speech disability, this service involves a CA who is specially trained in understanding a variety of speech disorders and repeats what the caller says in a manner that makes the caller's words clear and understandable to the called party. No special telephone is needed.
- **Shared Non-English Language Relay Services**. Due to the large number of Spanish speakers in the United States, the FCC requires interstate TRS providers to offer Spanish-to-Spanish traditional TRS. Although Spanish language relay is not required for intrastate TRS, many states with large numbers of Spanish speakers offer this service voluntarily. The FCC also allows TRS providers who voluntarily offer other shared non-English language interstate TRS, such as French-to-French, to be compensated from the federal TRS fund.
- **Captioned Telephone Service**. Used by persons with a hearing disability but some residual hearing. It uses a special telephone that has a text screen to display captions of what the other party to the conversation is saying. A captioned telephone allows the user, on one line, to speak to the called party and to simultaneously listen to the other party and read captions of what the other

Telecommunications Relay Service | 143

party is saying. There is a "two-line" version of captioned telephone service that offers additional features, such as call-waiting, *69, call forwarding, and direct dialing for 911 emergency service. Unlike traditional TRS, where the CA types what the called party says, the CA repeats or revoices what the called party says. Speech recognition technology automatically transcribes the CA's voice into text, which is then transmitted directly to the user's captioned telephone text display.

- **IP Captioned Telephone Service.** Combines elements of captioned telephone service and IP Relay. IP captioned telephone service can be provided in a variety of ways but uses the Internet—rather than the telephone network—to provide the link and captions between the caller with a hearing disability and the CA. It allows the user to simultaneously both listen to and read the text of what the other party in a telephone conversation is saying. IP captioned telephone service can be used with an existing voice telephone and a computer or other Web-enabled device without requiring any specialized equipment.
- **Internet Protocol Relay Service.** A text-based form of TRS that uses the Internet, rather than traditional telephone lines, for the leg of the call between the person with a hearing or speech disability and the CA. Otherwise, the call is generally handled just like a TTY-based TRS call. The user may use a computer or other web-enabled device to communicate with the CA. The FCC does not require IP Relay.
- **Video Relay Service (VRS).** This Internet-based form of TRS allows persons whose primary language is American Sign Language (ASL) to communicate with the CA in ASL using video conferencing equipment. The CA speaks what is signed to the called party, and signs the called party's response back to the caller. VRS is not required by the FCC but is offered by several TRS providers. VRS allows conversations to flow in near real-time and in a faster and more natural manner than text-based TRS. Beginning

January 1, 2006, TRS providers that offer VRS must provide it 24 hours a day, seven days a week, and must answer incoming calls within a specific period of time so that VRS users do not have to wait for a long time.

711 ACCESS TO TELECOMMUNICATIONS RELAY SERVICE

Just as you can call 411 for information, you can dial 711 to connect to certain forms of TRS anywhere in the United States. Dialing 711 makes it easier for travelers to use TRS because they do not have to remember TRS numbers in every state. 711 access is not available for CTS, IP CTS, VRS, or IP Relay.[1]

---

[1] "Telecommunications Relay Service," Federal Communications Commission (FCC), August 16, 2022. Available online. URL: www.fcc.gov/consumers/guides/telecommunications-relay-service-trs. Accessed August 10, 2024.

Part 4 | Protections, Rights, and Benefits

Chapter 21 | The Right to Effective Communication

MAKING COMMUNICATION ACCESSIBLE FOR PEOPLE WITH COMMUNICATION DISABILITIES

People who have vision, hearing, or speech disabilities (communication disabilities) use different ways to communicate. For example, people who are blind may give and receive information audibly rather than in writing, and people who are deaf may give and receive information through writing or sign language rather than through speech.

The Americans with Disabilities Act (ADA) requires that Title II entities (state and local governments) and Title III entities (businesses and nonprofit organizations that serve the public) communicate effectively with people who have communication disabilities. The goal is to ensure that communication with people with these disabilities is equally effective as communication with people without disabilities.

The purpose of the effective communication rules is to ensure that the person with a vision, hearing, or speech disability can communicate with, receive information from, and convey information to, the covered entity.

Covered entities must provide auxiliary aids and services when needed to communicate effectively with people with communication disabilities.

The key to communicating effectively is to consider the nature, length, complexity, and context of the communication and the person's normal method(s) of communication.

The rules apply to communicating with the person receiving the covered entity's goods or services and, in appropriate circumstances, with that person's parent, spouse, or companion.

EFFECTIVE COMMUNICATION PROVISIONS

Covered entities must provide aids and services when needed to communicate effectively with people with communication disabilities.

The key to deciding what aid or service is needed to communicate effectively is to consider the nature, length, complexity, and context of the communication and the person's normal method(s) of communication.

Some easy solutions work in relatively simple and straightforward situations. For example:
- In a retail setting, pointing to product information or writing notes back and forth to answer simple questions about a product may allow a person who is deaf to decide whether to purchase the product.
- In a lunchroom or restaurant, reading the menu to a person who is blind allows that person to decide what dish to order.

Other solutions may be needed where the information being communicated is more extensive or complex. For example:
- In a doctor's office, an interpreter is generally needed to take the medical history of a patient who uses sign language or to discuss a serious diagnosis and its treatment options.
- In a law firm, providing an accessible electronic copy of a legal document that is being drafted for a client who is blind allows the client to read the draft at home using a computer screen-reading program.

A person's method(s) of communication are also key. For example, sign language interpreters are effective only for people who use sign language. Other methods of communication, such as those described above, are needed for people who may have lost their hearing later in life and do not use sign language. Similarly, Braille is effective only for people who read Braille. Other methods are needed for people with vision disabilities who do not read Braille, such as providing accessible electronic text documents, forms, and so on, that the person's screen reader program can access.

Covered entities are also required to accept telephone calls placed through Telecommunications Relay Service (TRS) and Video Relay

The Right to Effective Communication | 149

Service (VRS), and staff who answer the telephone must treat relay calls like other calls. If necessary, the communications assistant will explain how the system works.

Remember, the purpose of the effective communication rules is to ensure that the person with a communication disability can receive information from and convey information to the covered entity.[1]

---

[1] ADA.gov, "ADA Requirements: Effective Communication," U.S. Department of Justice (DOJ), February 28, 2020. Available online. URL: www.ada.gov/resources/effective-communication. Accessed August 8, 2024.

Chapter 22 | Services for Students with Speech and Language Impairments

Many children are identified as having a speech or language impairment after entering the public school system. A teacher may notice difficulties in a child's speech or communication skills and refer the child for evaluation. Parents may also request to have their child evaluated. The public school system provides this evaluation free of charge.

If the child is found to have a disability under the Individuals with Disabilities Education Act (IDEA)—such as a speech-language impairment—school staff will work with the parents to develop an Individualized Education Program (IEP). The IEP is similar to an Individualized Family Service Plan (IFSP). It describes the child's unique needs and the services that have been designed to meet those needs. Special education and related services are provided at no cost to parents.

Communication skills are central to the educational experience. Eligible students with speech or language impairments should take advantage of the special education and related services available in public schools.

The types of support and services provided can vary greatly from student to student, just as speech-language impairments do. Special education and related services are planned and delivered based on each student's individualized educational and developmental needs.

Most, if not all, students with a speech or language impairment will require speech-language pathology services. This related service is defined by the Individuals with Disabilities Education Act (IDEA) as follows:

Speech-language pathology services include:
- identification of children with speech or language impairments
- diagnosis and appraisal of specific speech or language impairments
- referral for medical or other professional attention necessary for the habilitation of speech or language impairments
- provision of speech and language services for the habilitation or prevention of communicative impairments
- counseling and guidance of parents, children, and teachers regarding speech and language impairments

In addition to diagnosing the nature of a child's speech-language difficulties, speech-language pathologists (SLPs) also provide:
- individual therapy for the child
- consultation with the child's teacher about the most effective ways to facilitate the child's communication in the classroom setting
- close collaboration with the family to develop goals and techniques for effective therapy in class and at home

Speech and/or language therapy may continue throughout a student's school years, either in the form of direct therapy or on a consultant basis.

Assistive technology (AT) can also be highly beneficial to students, especially those whose physical conditions make communication difficult. Each student's IEP team must consider whether the student would benefit from AT, such as an electronic communication system or other devices. AT is often the key that helps students engage in the give and take of shared thought, complete their schoolwork, and demonstrate their learning.[1]

---

[1] "Speech and Language Impairments," U.S. Department of Education (ED), January 2011. Available online. URL: https://files.eric.ed.gov/fulltext/ED572698.pdf. Accessed August 8, 2024.

Chapter 23 | The Individuals with Disabilities Education Act (IDEA)

OVERVIEW OF INDIVIDUALS WITH DISABILITIES EDUCATION ACT

The Individuals with Disabilities Education Act (IDEA) is a law that ensures a free appropriate public education is available to eligible children with disabilities throughout the nation. It provides special education and related services to those children.

The IDEA governs how states and public agencies provide early intervention, special education, and related services to more than 8 million eligible infants, toddlers, children, and youth with disabilities (as of the school year 2022–2023).

EARLY INTERVENTION AND SPECIAL EDUCATION

Infants and toddlers—birth through age two—with disabilities and their families receive early intervention services under IDEA Part C. Children and youth aged 3 through 21 receive special education and related services under IDEA Part B.

PROGRAMS AUTHORIZED BY THE INDIVIDUALS WITH DISABILITIES EDUCATION ACT

The IDEA authorizes several key programs:

Office of Special Education Programs Formula Grant Programs

Office of Special Education Programs (OSEP) administers three formula grant programs authorized by the IDEA. These formula grants are awarded to states annually to support early intervention services for infants and toddlers with disabilities and their families, preschool children aged three through five, and special education for children and youth with disabilities.

Part B Formula Grants
- Assist states in providing a free appropriate public education in the least restrictive environment for children with disabilities, aged 3 through 21.
- Grants to States Program
  - Authorized by Part B, Section 611 for children aged 3 through 21.
- Preschool Grants Program
  - Authorized by Part B, Section 619 for children aged 3 through 5.

Part C Formula Grants
- Support early intervention services for infants and toddlers.
- Grants for Infants and Families Program
  - Authorized by Part C for infants and toddlers, birth through age two, and their families.

Discretionary Grants

The U.S. Department of Education awards these grants through a competitive process. The OSEP conducts application reviews through a formal peer review process using a standing panel. Reviewers score applications based on legislative and regulatory requirements and published selection criteria established for the grant programs and projects.

LEGISLATIVE BACKGROUND

Congress reauthorized the IDEA in 2004 and most recently amended it through Public Law 114-95, the Every Student Succeeds Act, in December 2015. In the law, Congress states:

> *Disability is a natural part of the human experience and in no way diminishes the right of individuals to participate*

The Individuals with Disabilities Education Act (IDEA)

in or contribute to society. Improving educational results for children with disabilities is an essential element of our national policy of ensuring equality of opportunity, full participation, independent living, and economic self-sufficiency for individuals with disabilities.

PURPOSE OF THE INDIVIDUALS WITH DISABILITIES EDUCATION ACT

The stated purpose of the IDEA is:
- to ensure that all children with disabilities have available to them a free appropriate public education that emphasizes special education and related services designed to meet their unique needs and prepare them for:
  - further education
  - employment
  - independent living
- to ensure that the rights of children with disabilities and parents of such children are protected
- to assist states, localities, educational service agencies, and federal agencies in providing for the education of all children with disabilities
- to assist states in the implementation of a statewide, comprehensive, coordinated, multidisciplinary, interagency system of early intervention services for infants and toddlers with disabilities and their families
- to ensure that educators and parents have the necessary tools to improve educational results for children with disabilities by supporting:
  - system improvement activities
  - coordinated research and personnel preparation
  - coordinated technical assistance, dissemination, and support
  - technology development and media services
- to assess and ensure the effectiveness of efforts to educate children with disabilities

The IDEA plays a crucial role in supporting the education and development of children with disabilities. Providing early intervention, special education, and related services ensures these children receive the support they need to achieve their full potential and lead independent, fulfilling lives.[1]

---

[1] "About IDEA," U.S. Department of Education (ED), December 15, 2015. Available online. URL: https://sites.ed.gov/idea/about-idea. Accessed August 7, 2024.

Chapter 24 | The Individualized Educational Plan (IEP)

WHAT IS AN INDIVIDUALIZED EDUCATION PROGRAM?

Each public school child who receives special education and related services must have an Individualized Education Program (IEP). Each IEP must be designed for one student and must be a truly individualized document. The IEP creates an opportunity for teachers, parents, school administrators, related services personnel, and students (when appropriate) to work together to improve educational results for children with disabilities. The IEP is the cornerstone of a quality education for each child with a disability.

PROCESS OF INDIVIDUALIZED EDUCATION PROGRAM
Step 1: Child Is Identified as Possibly Needing Special Education and Related Services

- **Child Find.** The state must identify, locate, and evaluate all children with disabilities in the state who need special education and related services. To do so, states conduct Child Find activities. A child may be identified by Child Find, and parents may be asked if the Child Find system can evaluate their child. Parents can also call the Child Find system and ask that their child be evaluated.
- **Referral or request for evaluation.** A school professional may ask that a child be evaluated to see if he or she has a disability. Parents may also contact the child's teacher or other school professional to ask that their child be evaluated. This request may be verbal or in writing. Parental consent is needed before the child may be evaluated. Evaluation needs

to be completed within a reasonable time after the parent gives consent.

Step 2: Child Is Evaluated

The evaluation must assess the child in all areas related to the child's suspected disability. The evaluation results will be used to decide the child's eligibility for special education and related services and to make decisions about an appropriate educational program for the child. If the parents disagree with the evaluation, they can take their child for an Independent Educational Evaluation (IEE) and ask that the school system pay for this IEE.

Step 3: Eligibility Is Decided

A group of qualified professionals and the parents look at the child's evaluation results. Together, they decide if the child is a "child with a disability," as defined by IDEA. Parents may ask for a hearing to challenge the eligibility decision.

Step 4: The Child Is Found Eligible for Services

If the child is found to be a "child with a disability," as defined by IDEA, he or she is eligible for special education and related services. Within 30 calendar days after a child is determined eligible, the IEP team must meet to write an IEP for the child.

Step 5: Individualized Education Program Meeting Is Scheduled

The school system schedules and conducts the IEP meeting. School staff must:
- contact the participants, including the parents
- notify parents early enough to make sure they have an opportunity to attend
- schedule the meeting at a time and place agreeable to parents and the school
- inform the parents of the purpose, time, and location of the meeting
- tell the parents who will be attending

The Individualized Educational Plan (IEP) | 159

- tell the parents that they may invite people to the meeting who have knowledge or special expertise about the child

Step 6: Individualized Education Program Meeting Is Held, and the Individualized Education Program Is Written

The IEP team gathers to discuss the child's needs and write the student's IEP. Parents and the student (when appropriate) are part of the team. If a different group decides the child's placement, the parents must be part of that group as well.

The parents must give consent before the school system may provide special education and related services to the child for the first time. The child begins to receive services as soon as possible after the meeting.

If the parents do not agree with the IEP and placement, they may discuss their concerns with other members of the IEP team and try to work out an agreement. If they still disagree, parents can ask for mediation, or the school may offer mediation. Parents may file a complaint with the state education agency and may request a due process hearing, at which time mediation must be available.

Step 7: Services Are Provided

The school ensures that the child's IEP is being carried out as it was written. Parents are given a copy of the IEP. Each of the child's teachers and service providers has access to the IEP and knows his or her specific responsibilities for carrying it out. This includes the accommodations, modifications, and supports that must be provided to the child in keeping with the IEP.

Step 8: Progress Is Measured and Reported to Parents

The child's progress toward the annual goals is measured, as stated in the IEP. His or her parents are regularly informed of their child's progress and whether that progress is enough for the child to achieve the goals by the end of the year. These progress reports must be given to parents at least as often as parents are informed of their nondisabled children's progress.

Step 9: Individualized Education Program Is Reviewed

The child's IEP is reviewed by the IEP team at least once a year, or more often if the parents or school ask for a review. If necessary, the IEP is revised. Parents, as team members, must be invited to attend these meetings. Parents can make suggestions for changes, agree or disagree with the IEP goals, and agree or disagree with the placement.

If parents do not agree with the IEP and placement, they may discuss their concerns with other members of the IEP team and try to work out an agreement. There are several options, including additional testing, an independent evaluation, asking for mediation (if available), or a due process hearing. They may also file a complaint with the state education agency.

Step 10: Child Is Reevaluated

The child must be reevaluated at least every three years. This evaluation is often called a "triennial." Its purpose is to determine whether the child continues to be a "child with a disability," as defined by IDEA, and what the child's educational needs are. However, the child must be reevaluated more often if conditions warrant or if the child's parent or teacher asks for a new evaluation.

If the child is blind or visually impaired, the IEP team shall provide for instruction in Braille or the use of Braille, unless it determines after an appropriate evaluation that the child does not need this instruction.[1]

---

[1] "A Guide to the Individualized Education Program," U.S. Department of Education (ED), August 30, 2019. Available online. URL: www2.ed.gov/parents/needs/speced/iepguide/index.html. Accessed August 8, 2024.

Chapter 25 | Legal Framework for Supporting Students with Communication Disabilities

FEDERAL REQUIREMENTS FOR PUBLIC SCHOOL STUDENTS WITH HEARING, VISION, OR SPEECH DISABILITIES

- Under the Individuals with Disabilities Education Act (IDEA), schools must provide a student with a disability a free appropriate public education (FAPE) designed to provide meaningful educational benefits through an Individualized Education Program (IEP).
- Under Title II of the Americans with Disabilities Act, schools must ensure, without charge, that communication with students with disabilities is as effective as communication with students without disabilities, giving primary consideration to students and parents in determining which auxiliary aids and services are necessary to provide such effective communication.

WILL THE AIDS AND SERVICES REQUIRED BE THE SAME UNDER FAPE AND TITLE II?

- It depends on the individual needs of the particular student.
- Sometimes the special education and related services provided to a student as part of FAPE under the IDEA will also meet the Title II requirements. In other instances, to meet the Title II requirements, a school might have to provide a student with aids or services that are not required by FAPE.

ARE SCHOOLS REQUIRED TO PROVIDE AID OR SERVICES AT THE PARENTS' REQUEST?

- Under Title II, the school must provide the aid or service requested unless the school can prove that a different auxiliary aid or service is as effective in meeting the student's communication needs (in which case the school must provide that alternative), or the school can prove that the aid or service would result in a fundamental alteration or in undue financial and administrative burdens (in which case the school must take other steps to ensure that the student can participate).
- Schools are not required to provide more aids or services than what is needed to ensure effective communication or to comply with requests about details of the aid or service (such as particular brands or models) that are not relevant to its effectiveness.

WHAT TYPES OF AIDS OR SERVICES MIGHT A STUDENT REQUIRE?

- There are no categorical rules. A school must assess the needs of each individual.
- For a student who is deaf, deaf-blind, or hard of hearing, some examples are the exchange of written materials, interpreters, note takers, real-time computer-aided transcription services (e.g., CART), assistive listening systems, accessible electronic and information technology, and open and closed captioning.
- For a student who is blind, deaf-blind, or has low vision, some examples are qualified readers, taped texts, audio recordings, Braille materials and refreshable Braille displays, accessible e-book readers, screen reader software, magnification software, optical readers, secondary auditory programs (SAP), and large print materials.
- For a student with a speech disability, some examples are a word or letter board, writing materials, spelling to

Legal Framework for Supporting Students | 163

communicate, a qualified sign language interpreter, a portable device that writes and/or produces speech, and telecommunications services.

MORE INFORMATION ABOUT THE RIGHTS OF STUDENTS WITH HEARING, VISION, OR SPEECH DISABILITIES

- The U.S. Department of Education's Office for Civil Rights (OCR) and Office of Special Education and Rehabilitative Services, along with the U.S. Department of Justice (DOJ), have issued a Dear Colleague Letter and a Frequently Asked Questions document explaining what federal law requires of schools to meet the communication needs of students with hearing, vision, or speech disabilities.

WHAT PARENTS CAN DO WHEN A CHILD'S EDUCATIONAL NEEDS ARE UNMET

- Arrange to meet with the IEP or 504 team or the school's Title II or 504 Coordinator.
- Consider using the school district's published disability grievance procedures.
- Under the IDEA, a parent challenging the provision of FAPE may request mediation, file a complaint with the State educational agency, or file a due process complaint to request an impartial administrative hearing.
- Under Title II, a parent may choose to file a lawsuit in court. Parents of an IDEA-eligible student generally must exhaust the administrative hearing procedures of the IDEA, which means obtaining a final decision under the IDEA's impartial due process hearing procedures, before filing a lawsuit seeking a remedy that is also available under the IDEA.
- OCR and DOJ both investigate complaints of disability discrimination at schools.
  - To learn how to file a complaint with OCR, call 800-421-3481 (TDD: 800-877-8339), email: ocr@ed.gov, or visit www.ed.gov/ocr/complaintintro.html.

- To learn how to file a complaint with DOJ, call 800-514-0301 (TTY: 800-514-0383), email ADA.complaint@usdoj.gov, or visit www.ada.gov/fact_on_complaint.htm.[1]

---

[1] "Meeting the Communication Needs of Students with Hearing, Vision, or Speech Disabilities," U.S. Department of Education (ED), November 12, 2014. Available online. URL: www2.ed.gov/about/offices/list/ocr/docs/dcl-factsheet-parent-201411.pdf. Accessed August 10, 2024.

Chapter 26 | Telecommunications Access for People with Disabilities

Federal Communications Commission (FCC) rules under Section 255 of the Communications Act require telecommunications equipment manufacturers and service providers to make their products and services accessible to people with disabilities if such access is readily achievable. Where access is not readily achievable, manufacturers and service providers must make their devices and services compatible with peripheral devices and specialized customer premises equipment commonly used by people with disabilities if such compatibility is readily achievable.

PRODUCTS AND SERVICES COVERED UNDER SECTION 255

Federal Communications Commission rules cover all hardware and software telephone network equipment and telecommunications equipment used in the home or office. Such equipment includes telephones, wireless handsets, fax machines, answering machines, and pagers.

FCC rules also cover basic and special telecommunications services, including regular telephone calls, call waiting, speed dialing, call forwarding, computer-provided directory assistance, call monitoring, caller identification, call tracing, repeat dialing, voice mail, and interactive voice response systems that provide callers with menus of choices.

IDENTIFYING ACCESS NEEDS

Companies should engage in several activities to identify barriers to accessibility and usability. For example:
- Companies should include individuals with disabilities in target groups for market research, product design, testing, pilot demonstrations, and product trials.
- Companies should work cooperatively with disability-related organizations.
- Companies should undertake reasonable efforts to test access solutions with people with disabilities.

WHEN MUST MANUFACTURERS AND SERVICE PROVIDERS EVALUATE ACCESS NEEDS?

Manufacturers and service providers must evaluate the accessibility, usability, and compatibility of their equipment and services as early and consistently as possible throughout their design, development, and manufacture. In addition, companies must review their products for accessibility at every "natural opportunity," including when they redesign products, upgrade services, or significantly change the way they group together product and service packages. Cosmetic changes that do not alter the product's actual design may not trigger the need to reevaluate access.

DO COMPANIES NEED TO REVIEW ALL THEIR PRODUCTS AND SERVICES FOR ACCESSIBILITY AND USABILITY?

Yes. Accessibility and usability must be assessed for individual products and services. Accessibility features that can be incorporated into the design of products or services with little or no difficulty or expense must be included in every product or service.

HOW WILL THE FCC DETERMINE WHICH ACTIONS ARE READILY ACHIEVABLE?

The "readily achievable" standard requires companies to incorporate access features that are easily accomplishable without much difficulty or expense. In determining what is readily achievable, companies must balance the costs and nature of the access required with their available resources. Companies with greater resources will need to do more to achieve access than companies with smaller budgets.

The FCC will make readily achievable determinations on a case-by-case basis.

IS NETWORK ARCHITECTURE COVERED BY THE FCC'S SECTION 255 RULES?

In addition to covering equipment and services, the FCC's rules require network architecture to be designed to facilitate access for people with disabilities. Network architecture covers the public switched telephone network and includes hardware or software databases associated with routing telecommunications services.

WHAT CAN YOU DO IF YOU ARE CONCERNED ABOUT THE ACCESSIBILITY OF AN ADVANCED COMMUNICATIONS PRODUCT OR SERVICE?

If you are concerned about the accessibility of an advanced communications product or service, you may want to contact the equipment manufacturer or service provider. You can find company contact information on the FCC website, by emailing dro@fcc.gov, or by calling 202-418-2517 (voice) or 844-432-2275 (videophone).[1]

---

[1] "Telecommunications Access for People with Disabilities," Federal Communications Commission (FCC), January 27, 2021. Available online. URL: www.fcc.gov/consumers/guides/telecommunications-access-people-disabilities. Accessed August 11, 2024.

Chapter 27 | Social Security Disability Programs

Chapter Contents
Section 27.1—Benefits for People with Disabilities......................170
Section 27.2—Benefits for Children with Disabilities.....................172
Section 27.3—Qualifying for Social Security Disability Benefits............176

Section 27.1 | Benefits for People with Disabilities

Social Security provides a source of income when you retire or if you cannot work due to a disability. Learn how you may be eligible for benefits through Social Security Disability Insurance (SSDI) or Supplemental Security Income (SSI) if you have a disability or are 65 or older.

DIFFERENCE BETWEEN SOCIAL SECURITY DISABILITY INSURANCE AND SUPPLEMENTAL SECURITY INCOME

Social Security Disability Insurance is tied to your work history. It pays benefits to you and certain members of your family if you:
- have a disability
- worked enough years to qualify and paid Social Security taxes during the years you worked

SSI does not require you to have a work history. It provides you with money to cover basics such as food, clothing, and housing if you are 65 or older or have a disability.

FIND OUT IF YOU ARE ELIGIBLE FOR SOCIAL SECURITY DISABILITY INSURANCE AND APPLY

Your eligibility for SSDI is based on your age, disability, and how long you worked. To find out if you are eligible for SSDI, use the Benefit Eligibility Screening Tool (www.ssa.gov/prepare/check-eligibility-for-benefits).

Your spouse or former spouse and your children may be eligible for benefits when you start receiving SSDI. Learn about family benefits and see if your family members may qualify (www.ssa.gov/family).

You have options to apply online, by phone, or in person.

If your application is approved, there will be a five-month waiting period for benefits to start. Learn how to appeal if your SSDI application is denied through this web page: www.ssa.gov/disability#anchor2.

FIND OUT IF YOU ARE ELIGIBLE FOR SUPPLEMENTAL SECURITY INCOME AND APPLY

Supplemental Security Income is for people who have little to no income and have a disability or are 65 or older.

Use the Benefit Eligibility Screening Tool to see if you are eligible for SSI (www.ssa.gov/prepare/check-eligibility-for-benefits).

You have options to apply online, by phone, or in person.
- To apply for SSI for a child, you can start the process online (www.ssa.gov/ssi) but must complete it either in person or by phone.
- Understand how to appeal a decision if your SSI application is denied from this web page: www.ssa.gov/ssi/text-appeals-ussi.htm.

WHEN ARE SOCIAL SECURITY DISABILITY INSURANCE AND SUPPLEMENTAL SECURITY INCOME BENEFITS PAID?

The day you receive your SSDI or SSI benefits each month is based on your birthdate.

If your payment is more than three days late, contact the Social Security Administration (SSA; https://faq.ssa.gov/en-us/Topic/article/KA-02423).

GET HELP WITH SECURITY DISABILITY INSURANCE AND SUPPLEMENTAL SECURITY INCOME BENEFITS

You can create a free "my Social Security" account to manage your benefits online (www.ssa.gov/onlineservices) and:
- Check on your application status.
- Update your name, address, and other information.
- Set up or change your direct deposit information to receive your benefits.
- Get tax documents to report income from SSDI benefits (SSI benefits are not taxable).
- Get a benefit verification letter to show what benefits you receive.

If you have specific questions:
- Review the SSA's frequently asked questions pages for SSDI (https://faq.ssa.gov/en-US/Topic/?id=CAT-01089) and SSI (https://faq.ssa.gov/en-US/topic/?id=CAT-01094).
- Contact the SSA directly (www.ssa.gov/agency/contact).[1]

Section 27.2 | Benefits for Children with Disabilities

ELIGIBILITY FOR SUPPLEMENTAL SECURITY INCOME AND SOCIAL SECURITY DISABILITY INSURANCE

Parents, caregivers, or representatives of children under 18 with disabilities that may make them eligible for Supplemental Security Income (SSI) payments can benefit from the following information. It is also relevant for adults with disabilities since childhood (before age 22) who might be entitled to Social Security Disability Insurance (SSDI) benefits. The SSDI benefit is called a "child's benefit" because it is paid on a parent's Social Security earnings record.

SUPPLEMENTAL SECURITY INCOME PAYMENTS FOR CHILDREN WITH DISABILITIES

The SSI provides monthly payments to people with limited income and resources who are 65 or older, blind, or disabled. Children under 18 are eligible if they have a medical condition or combination of conditions that meets Social Security's definition of disability. Their income and resources must fall within the eligibility limits. The amount of the SSI payment differs from state to state because some states add to the SSI payment. Your local Social Security office can provide more information about your state's total SSI payment.

---

[1] "SSDI and SSI Benefits for People with Disabilities," USA.gov, July 16, 2024. Available online. URL: www.usa.gov/social-security-disability. Accessed August 9, 2024.

INCOME AND RESOURCE RULES FOR SUPPLEMENTAL SECURITY INCOME

The SSI eligibility considers a child's income and resources, as well as those of family members living in the household. These rules apply if your child lives at home or is away at school but returns home periodically and is subject to your control. If the income and resources exceed the allowed amount, the child's application for SSI payments will be denied. SSI payments are limited to $30 monthly when children are in a medical facility and health insurance covers their care.

DISABILITY RULES FOR SUPPLEMENTAL SECURITY INCOME

To be considered medically eligible for SSI, a child must meet the following requirements:

- A child who is not blind must not be working or earning more than $1,550 a month in 2024, and a child who is blind must not be working or earning more than $2,590.
- The child must have a medical condition or a combination of conditions that result in "marked and severe functional limitations," meaning the condition(s) must very seriously limit the child's activities.
- The condition(s) must be disabling or expected to be disabling for at least 12 months, or be expected to result in death.

PROVIDING INFORMATION ABOUT YOUR CHILD'S CONDITION

When applying for SSI payments for your child based on a disability, detailed information about the child's medical condition and its effect on daily activities will be required. Permission will be needed to obtain information from doctors, teachers, therapists, and other professionals. Providing medical or school records will help expedite the decision-making process.

WHAT HAPPENS NEXT?

The information provided will be sent to the Disability Determination Services office in your state, where doctors and trained staff will review it. If necessary, they may request additional medical examinations or tests, which the agency will pay for.

IMMEDIATE SUPPLEMENTAL SECURITY INCOME PAYMENTS FOR CERTAIN CONDITIONS

The SSI payments may be made immediately for up to six months for certain medical conditions while the state agency decides on eligibility. Conditions that may qualify for immediate payments include total blindness, total deafness, cerebral palsy (CP), Down syndrome, muscular dystrophy, severe intellectual disability (for children aged 4 or older), symptomatic HIV infection, and birth weight below 2 pounds, 10 ounces.

SUPPLEMENTAL SECURITY INCOME DISABILITY REVIEWS

After receiving SSI, a child's medical condition must be reviewed periodically to ensure continued eligibility. Reviews are conducted:
- every three years for children whose conditions are expected to improve or for which improvement is possible
- by age one for babies receiving SSI due to low birth weight

TRANSITION TO ADULT SUPPLEMENTAL SECURITY INCOME AT AGE 18

At age 18, different medical and nonmedical rules apply for SSI eligibility. The income and resources of family members are not considered, except for a spouse. A review using adult disability rules will determine continued eligibility.

SOCIAL SECURITY DISABILITY INSURANCE BENEFITS FOR ADULTS WITH DISABILITIES SINCE CHILDHOOD

The SSDI program pays benefits to adults with disabilities that began before age 22, based on a parent's Social Security earnings record. To qualify, a parent must be receiving Social Security retirement or disability benefits, or have died after working enough to be eligible for Social Security benefits. SSDI benefits continue if the individual has a disability, though marriage may affect eligibility.

DETERMINING SOCIAL SECURITY DISABILITY INSURANCE ELIGIBILITY

For adults over 18, disability is evaluated using adult criteria. Applications are sent to the state's Disability Determination Services for evaluation.

APPLYING FOR SUPPLEMENTAL SECURITY INCOME OR SOCIAL SECURITY DISABILITY INSURANCE BENEFITS

To apply for SSI or SSDI, you must complete an application and a Child Disability Report. This report collects information about the disabling condition and its effect on the child's ability to function. Applications can be started online, by phone, or in person. Providing detailed medical information and records will aid in the determination process.

EMPLOYMENT SUPPORT PROGRAMS FOR YOUNG PEOPLE WITH DISABILITIES

Supplemental Security Income and SSDI recipients can access various programs that encourage employment, such as excluding most of a student's income when calculating SSI payments, Plans to Achieve Self-Support (PASS), and continued Medicaid coverage despite high earnings. SSDI beneficiaries can also receive help with work expenses and vocational training.

MEDICAID AND MEDICARE

Medicaid provides health care for those with limited income and resources. In most states, children receiving SSI automatically qualify for Medicaid. Medicare is available to those who have received SSDI for at least two years or meet specific conditions like End-Stage Renal Disease or Amyotrophic Lateral Sclerosis.

CHILDREN'S HEALTH INSURANCE PROGRAM

Children's Health Insurance Program (CHIP) provides health insurance to children from working families with incomes too high for Medicaid but too low for private insurance. It covers prescription drugs, vision, hearing, and mental health services.

OTHER HEALTH-CARE SERVICES

Children receiving SSI may be referred to services under the Children with Special Health Care Needs provision of the Social Security Act. These services, managed by state health agencies, provide various health services through clinics, private offices, hospitals, or community agencies.[1]

Section 27.3 | Qualifying for Social Security Disability Benefits

SOCIAL SECURITY DISABILITY INSURANCE BENEFITS

To qualify for Social Security Disability Insurance (SSDI) benefits, individuals must:
- have worked in jobs covered by Social Security
- have a medical condition that meets Social Security's strict definition of disability

In general, monthly benefits are paid to individuals who are unable to work for a year or more because of a disability. Typically, there is a five-month waiting period, and the first benefit is paid the sixth full month after the date the disability began.

Social Security may pay disability benefits for up to 12 months before the application if it is found that the individual had a disability during that time and meets all other requirements.

Benefits usually continue until the individual can work again on a regular basis. There are also several special rules, known as "work incentives," that provide continued benefits and health care coverage to help individuals transition back to work.

If individuals are receiving SSDI benefits when they reach full retirement age, their disability benefits automatically convert to retirement benefits, but the amount remains the same.

---

[1] "Benefits for Children with Disabilities," U.S. Social Security Administration (SSA), January 2024. Available online. URL: www.ssa.gov/pubs/EN-05-10026.pdf. Accessed August 11, 2024.

HOW MUCH WORK DO YOU NEED?

In addition to meeting the definition of disability, individuals must have worked long enough—and recently enough—under Social Security to qualify for disability benefits.

Social Security work credits are based on total yearly wages or self-employment income. Individuals can earn up to four credits each year. For example, in 2024, one earns one credit for each $1,730 in wages or self-employment income. When one has earned $6,920, they have earned four credits for the year.

The number of work credits needed to qualify for disability benefits depends on the age when the disability begins. Generally, 40 credits are needed, 20 of which were earned in the last 10 years ending with the year the disability begins. However, younger workers may qualify with fewer credits.

DISABILITY DEFINITION

The definition of disability under Social Security differs from that of other programs. Only total disability is eligible for benefits—no benefits are payable for partial disability or short-term disability.

An individual is considered to have a qualifying disability under Social Security rules if:
- They cannot perform work at the Substantial Gainful Activity (SGA) level because of a medical condition.
- They cannot perform work they did previously or adjust to other work because of their medical condition.
- Their condition has lasted or is expected to last for at least one year or to result in death.

This is a strict definition of disability. The Social Security program rules assume that working families have access to other resources to provide financial support during periods of short-term disabilities, such as workers' compensation, insurance, savings, and investments.

DECISION ON QUALIFYING DISABILITY

If an individual has enough work to qualify for disability benefits, a step-by-step process involving five questions is used to determine if they have a qualifying disability:

Are You Working?

Earnings guidelines are used to evaluate whether work activity is SGA. If an individual is working in 2024 and their earnings average more than $1,550 per month ($2,590 if blind), they generally cannot be considered to have a disability.

Is Your Condition Severe?

The condition must significantly limit the ability to perform basic work-related activities for at least 12 months. If it does not, it is determined that there is no qualifying disability.

Is Your Condition Found on the List of Disabling Conditions?

For each of the major body systems, there is a list of medical conditions considered severe enough to prevent a person from doing SGA. If a condition is not on the list, it is assessed whether it is as severe as a condition on the list.

Can You Do the Work You Did Previously?

It is decided whether medical impairments prevent an individual from performing any of their past work. If not, it is determined that there is no qualifying disability.

Can You Do Any Other Type of Work?

If an individual cannot do the work they did in the past, it is assessed whether there is other work they could do despite their medical impairments, considering their medical conditions, age, education, past work experience, and any transferable skills they may have. If they cannot do other work, they qualify for disability benefits. If they can do other work, the claim is denied.[1]

---

[1] "How You Qualify," U.S. Social Security Administration (SSA), March 14, 2015. Available online. URL: www.ssa.gov/benefits/disability/qualify.html. Accessed August 9, 2024.

Part 5 | Additional Resources

Chapter 28 | Directory of Organizations Providing Support for People with Communication Disabilities

Americans with Disabilities Act (ADA)
950 Pennsylvania Ave., N.W.
Washington, DC 20530-0001
Toll-Free: 800-514-0301
Toll-Free TTY: 833-610-1264
Website: www.ada.gov

Centers for Disease Control and Prevention (CDC)
1600 Clifton Rd., N.E.
Atlanta, GA 30329
Toll-Free: 800-CDC-INFO (800-232-4636)
Phone: 770-488-1725
Toll-Free TTY: 888-232-6348
Website: www.cdc.gov
Email: hrcs@cdc.gov

***Eunice Kennedy Shriver* National Institute of Child Health and Human Development (NICHD)**
P.O. Box 3006
Rockville, MD 20847
Toll-Free: 800-370-2943
Website: www.nichd.nih.gov
Email: NICHDInformationResourceCenter@mail.nih.gov

Resources in this chapter were compiled from several sources deemed reliable; all contact information was verified and updated in September 2024.

Federal Communications Commission (FCC)
45 L St., N.E.
Washington, DC 20554
Toll-Free: 888-CALL-FCC (888-225-5322)
Phone: 202-418-1122
Toll-Free TTY: 888-TELL-FCC (888-835-5322)
Toll-Free Fax: 866-418-0232
Website: www.fcc.gov

MedlinePlus
8600 Rockville Pike
Bethesda, MD 20894
Toll-Free: 888-FIND-NLM (888-346-3656)
Phone: 301-594-5983
Website: www.medlineplus.gov

National Council on Disability (NCD)
1331 F St., N.W., Ste. 850
Washington, DC 20004
Phone: 202-272-2004
Fax: 202-272-2022
Website: www.ncd.gov
Email: ncd@ncd.gov

National Eye Institute (NEI)
31 Center Dr., MSC 2510
Bethesda, MD 20892-2510
Phone: 301-496-5248
Website: www.nei.nih.gov
Email: 2020@nei.nih.gov

National Institute on Aging (NIA)
P.O. Box 8057
Gaithersburg, MD 20898
Toll-Free: 800-222-2225
Website: www.nia.nih.gov
Email: niaic@nia.nih.gov

National Institute on Deafness and Other Communication Disorders (NIDCD)
1 Communication Ave.
Bethesda, MD 20892-3456
Toll-Free: 800-241-1044
Toll-Free TTY: 800-241-1055
Website: www.nidcd.nih.gov
Email: nidcdinfo@nidcd.nih.gov

Ready.gov
500 C St., S.W.
Washington, DC 20472
Toll-Free: 800-621-FEMA (800-621-3362)
Website: www.ready.gov
Email: fema-news-desk@fema.dhs.gov

U.S. Agency for International Development (USAID)
1300 Pennsylvania Ave., N.W.
Washington DC 20004
Toll-Free: 800-996-7566
Phone: 202-712-0000
Website: www.usaid.gov

U.S. Department of Education (ED)
400 Maryland Ave., S.W.
Washington, DC 20202
Toll-Free: 800-USA-LEARN (800-872-5327)
Phone: 202-401-2000
Website: www.ed.gov

U.S. Department of Health and Human Services (HHS)
200 Independence Ave., S.W.
Washington, DC 20201
Toll-Free: 877-696-6775
Website: www.hhs.gov

U.S. Department of Labor (DOL)
200 Constitution Ave., N.W.
Washington, DC 20210
Toll-Free: 866-4-USA-DOL (866-487-2365)
Website: www.dol.gov

U.S. Department of Transportation (DOT)
1200 New Jersey Ave., S.E.
Washington, DC 20590
Toll-Free: 855-368-4200
Phone: 202-366-4000
Website: www.transportation.gov

U.S. Department of Veterans Affairs (VA)
810 Vermont Ave., N.W.
Washington, DC 20420
Toll-Free: 800-698-2411
Website: www.va.gov

U.S. Food and Drug Administration (FDA)
10903 New Hampshire Ave.
Silver Spring, MD 20993
Toll-Free: 888-INFO-FDA (888-463-6332)
Phone: 301-796-8240
Website: www.fda.gov

U.S. Social Security Administration (SSA)
P.O. Box 17769
Baltimore, MD 21235-7769
Toll-Free: 800-772-1213
Toll-Free TTY: 800-325-0778
Website: www.ssa.gov

INDEX

INDEX

Page numbers followed by "n" refer to citation information; by "t" indicate tables; and by "f" indicate figures.

A

AAC *see* augmentative and alternative communication
abductor spasmodic dysphonia, defined 28
ABR *see* auditory brainstem response
acquired apraxia of speech *see* apraxia of speech
ADA.gov
    publication
        ADA requirements: effective communication 149n
adductor spasmodic dysphonia, defined 28
age-related hearing loss, defined 49
aging
    hearing aids 114
    hearing disorders 48
    low vision 52
    people with disabilities 87
ALDs *see* assistive listening devices
alternative modes, language acquisition 12
American Sign Language (ASL)
    communication barriers 80
    described 104
    overview 109–111
    video relay service (VRS) 143
Americans with Disabilities Act (ADA), contact information 181
AOS *see* apraxia of speech
aphasia
    apraxia of speech (AOS) 33
    neurodegenerative disorders 13
    overview 60–62
apraxia of speech (AOS)
    aphasia 60
    language disorder 6
    overview 32–35
ASL *see* American Sign Language
assistive device
    described 111
    residual hearing 105
    spasmodic dysphonia 30
assistive listening devices (ALDs), defined 112
audiologist
    audiology evaluation 99
    auditory processing disorder (APD) 56
    hearing aid 115
    hearing loss 51
    language disorders 6
    speech-language pathologists (SLPs) 123
auditory brainstem response (ABR), defined 100
auditory processing disorder (APD) *see* central auditory processing disorder (CAPD)
auditory-oral program, defined 107
auditory-verbal program, defined 108
augmentative and alternative communication (AAC)
    assistive devices 112
    language acquisition 12

autism spectrum disorder (ASD)
    overview 65–67
    speech-language therapy 126

B
behavioral audiometry evaluation, described 100
bilingual program, defined 108
brain and sensory integration, described 11
brain injuries, neurogenic stuttering 37

C
CAPD *see* central auditory processing disorder
CASE *see* Conceptually Accurate Signed English
Centers for Disease Control and Prevention (CDC)
    contact information 181
    publications
        building communication skills 109n
        cleft lip/cleft palate 65n
        communication 5n
        hearing loss communication methods 107n
        screening for hearing loss 101n
        treatment and intervention for hearing loss 98n
central auditory processing disorder (CAPD), overview 55–57
Child Find, Individualized Education Program (IEP) 157
childhood apraxia of speech (CAS) *see* apraxia of speech
children
    apraxia of speech (AOS) 32
    central auditory processing disorder (CAPD) 55
    children with disabilities 172
    developmental communication disorders 12

developmental language disorder (DLD) 40
early intervention services 95
hearing loss 48
language impairments 152
learning disabilities 129
orofacial clefts 63
social barriers 82
speech and language development 5
speechreading 107
cleft lip, depicted 63
cleft palate
    depicted 64
    speech-language pathologists (SLPs) 123
cochlear implant
    assistive listening devices (ALDs) 112
    hearing loss 104
    overview 116–119
Conceptually Accurate Signed English (CASE)
    defined 104
    developing communication skills 109
cued speech, defined 104

D
developmental language disorder (DLD)
    communication disorders 17
    overview 40–42
    specific language impairment (SLI) 43
    speech disorder 6
developmental stuttering
    communication disorders 17
    stuttering 37
disability disclosure 83
disaster preparedness, people with disabilities 135
disfluent speech *see* stuttering

DLD *see* developmental language disorder
dysarthria
   aphasia 60
   apraxia of speech (AOS) 32
   neurodegenerative disorders 13

E

early communication, described 3
Early Hearing Detection and Intervention (EHDI) 96, 98
early intervention
   financial assistance 116
   Individuals with Disabilities Education Act (IDEA) 153
   learning disabilities 130
   overview 94–98
EHDI *see* Early Hearing Detection and Intervention
employment
   disability disclosure 84
   Individuals with Disabilities Education Act (IDEA) 155
   support programs 175
Eunice Kennedy Shriver National Institute of Child Health and Human Development (NICHD)
   contact information 181
   publications
      learning disabilities 131n
      speech-language therapy for autism 127n

F

FAPE *see* free appropriate public education
FCC *see* Federal Communications Commission
Federal Communications Commission (FCC)
   contact information 182
   publications
      Speech to Speech (STS) relay service 139n
      telecommunications access for people with disabilities 167n
      Telecommunications Relay Service (TRS) 144n
   Speech to Speech (STS) relay service 138
   telecommunications access 165
finger spelling
   American Sign Language (ASL) 104, 110
   bilingual program 108
   defined 105
   Manually Coded English (MCE) 106
free appropriate public education (FAPE), Individuals with Disabilities Education Act (IDEA) 153, 161

G

gastroesophageal reflux disease (GERD)
   described 25
   voice problem 21
genetic factors
   childhood apraxia of speech (CAS) 33
   developmental stuttering 37
GERD *see* gastroesophageal reflux disease

H

hearing aids, overview 114–116
hearing loss
   assistive listening devices (ALDs) 112
   audiologist 56
   auditory processing disorder (APD) 55
   developmental language disorder (DLD) 40
   early intervention 97
   family support services 98
   hearing aids 114
   language and literacy 13

hearing loss, *continued*
   learning language 97
   overview 48–51
   screening 98
   specific language impairment (SLI) 43
hoarseness
   overview 23–27
   vocal fold paralysis 31

I

IDEA *see* Individuals with Disabilities Education Act
IEE *see* Independent Educational Evaluation
IEP *see* Individualized Education Program
IFSP *see* Individualized Family Service Plan
Independent Educational Evaluation (IEE) 158
Individualized Education Program (IEP)
   disability disclosure 83
   overview 151–160
Individualized Family Service Plan (IFSP) 151
Individuals with Disabilities Education Act (IDEA)
   disability disclosure 83
   federal requirements 161
   overview 153–156
   students 151
interventions 129

L

language
   apraxia of speech (AOS) 33
   auditory processing disorder (APD) 56
   autism spectrum disorder (ASD) 67
   brain and sensory integration 12
   communication barriers 81
   communication disabilities 163
   communication techniques 104
   defined 3
   developmental language disorder (DLD) 41
   hearing loss 97
   speech-language pathologists (SLPs) 122
   speech-language therapy 126
   Telecommunications Relay Service (TRS) 142
language acquisition
   American Sign Language (ASL) 110
   brain and sensory integration 12
language and literacy 13
language delay, developmental language disorder (DLD) 40
language disorder
   apraxia of speech (AOS) 33
   assistive devices 111
   autism spectrum disorder (ASD) 66
   language acquisition 12
   speech and language development 6
   speech-language pathologist (SLP) 29, 123
language statistics 17
laryngeal dystonia *see* spasmodic dysphonia
laryngeal papillomatosis
   vocal fold paralysis 27
   voice problems 21
laryngectomy, speech disabilities 137
laryngitis, defined 25
learning disabilities
   apraxia of speech (AOS) 33
   overview 129–130
lipreading *see* speechreading
literacy, hearing loss 13
low birth weight
   overview 67–69
   Supplemental Security Income (SSI) 174
low vision
   communication disabilities 162
   overview 51–53
Lyme disease, vocal fold paralysis 24

M

MedlinePlus, contact information 182
mental health
   avoiding offensive language 78
   Children's Health Insurance Program (CHIP) 175
mixed spasmodic dysphonia, defined 28
multiple sclerosis (MS)
   people-first language 78
   vocal fold paralysis 26

N

National Center on Birth Defects and Developmental Disabilities (NCBDDD)
   publications
      acting early 95n
      common barriers to participation 82n
      communicating with and about people with disabilities 78n
      disability and health information for family caregivers 135n
      early intervention 96n
National Council on Disability (NCD), contact information 182
National Eye Institute (NEI)
   contact information 182
   publication
      low vision 53n
National Institute on Aging (NIA)
   contact information 182
   publication
      hearing loss in older adults 51n
National Institute on Deafness and Other Communication Disorders (NIDCD)
   contact information 183
   publications
      American Sign Language (ASL) 111n
      aphasia 62n
      apraxia of speech (AOS) 35n
      assistive devices 113n
      autism spectrum disorder 67n
      cochlear implants 117n
      developmental language disorder 42n
      hearing aids 116n
      hoarseness 27n
      low birth weight and communication problems 69n
      NIDCD strategic plan 2017–2021 14n
      quick statistics about voice, speech, and language 17n
      spasmodic dysphonia 30n
      specific language impairment 45n
      speech and language developmental milestones 9n
      stuttering 40n
      taking care of your voice 23n
      vocal fold paralysis 32n
      voice, speech, and language 3n
natural gestures
   defined 106
   developing communication skills 109
neurodegenerative disorders, communication disorders 14
neurogenic stuttering, defined 37
neurologist, defined 29

O

OAE *see* otoacoustic emissions
OM *see* otitis media
orofacial clefts
   overview 62–65
   see also cleft lip; cleft palate
otitis media (OM), hearing loss 50
otoacoustic emissions (OAE), defined 100
otolaryngologist
   behavioral audiometry evaluation 101
   spasmodic dysphonia 29
   voice health 21

P

Parkinson disease (PD), vocal fold paralysis 30
people-first language, overview 77–78
phonological disorders, statistics 16
presbycusis *see* age-related hearing loss

Q

QOL *see* quality of life
quality of life (QOL)
   speech-language pathologist (SPL) 124
   stereotyping 79
   stuttering 36

R

Ready.gov, contact information 183
recurrent respiratory papillomatosis (RRP), hoarseness 27
residual hearing
   bilingual program 108
   captioned telephone service 142
   listening/auditory training 105
   spoken speech 106
RRP *see* recurrent respiratory papillomatosis

S

service animal, communication disabilities 73
SLI *see* specific language impairment
SLP *see* speech-language pathologist
social interaction
   autism spectrum disorder (ASD) 65
   defined 127
Social Security Disability Insurance (SSDI), people with disabilities 170
spasmodic dysphonia
   defined 16
   overview 27–30
   voice problems 21
special education
   early intervention services 96
   hearing loss 69
   Individualized Education Program (IEP) 157
   language impairments 151
   speech disabilities 163
specific language impairment (SLI)
   developmental communication disorders 12
   developmental language disorder (DLD) 40
   overview 43–45
speech disorder
   aphasia 60
   communication disorders 16
   language development 6
   stuttering 36
   Telecommunications Relay Service (TRS) 137
speech pathology, speech therapy 124
speech sound disorders
   apraxia of speech (AOS) 32
   communication disorders 16
speech statistics 16
Speech to Speech (STS), overview 137–139
speech-generating devices, communication devices 113
speech-language pathologist (SLP)
   auditory processing disorder (APD) 56
   autism spectrum disorder (ASD) 66
   cochlear implants 117
   developmental language disorder (DLD) 41
   hoarseness 25
   language disorder 6
   language impairments 152
   overview 122–123
   residual hearing 105
   vocal fold paralysis 31

speechreading
   auditory-oral program 108
   cued speech 105
   described 106
SSDI *see* Social Security Disability Insurance
SSI *see* Supplemental Security Income
stammering *see* stuttering
statistics, overview 15–17
STS *see* Speech to Speech
stuttering, overview 36–40
stuttering therapy 39
sudden deafness *see* sudden hearing loss
sudden hearing loss, defined 48
sudden sensorineural hearing loss *see* sudden hearing loss
Supplemental Security Income (SSI), overview 171–176
swallowing disorders, speech-language pathologist (SLP) 122
swallowing statistics 17
synthetic speech, spasmodic dysphonia 29

T

Telecommunications Relay Service (TRS), overview 141–144
telehealth 125
throat disorders, vocal fold paralysis 31
thyroid problems, hoarseness 27
tinnitus, described 49
TRS *see* Telecommunications Relay Service

U

U.S. Agency for International Development (USAID), contact information 183
U.S. Bureau of Labor Statistics (BLS)
   publication
      speech-language pathologists 123n
U.S. Department of Education (ED)
   contact information 183
   publications
      auditory processing disorders 57n
      communication needs of students with hearing, vision, or speech disabilities 164n
      IDEA (Individuals with Disabilities Education Act) 156n
      Individualized Education Program (IEP) 160n
      speech and language impairments 152n
U.S. Department of Health and Human Services (HHS), contact information 183
U.S. Department of Homeland Security (DHS)
   publication
      interacting with people who have disabilities 76n
U.S. Department of Labor (DOL)
   contact information 184
   publications
      people with disabilities and business goals 89n
      youth, disclosure, and the workplace 86n
U.S. Department of Transportation (DOT), contact information 184
U.S. Department of Veterans Affairs (VA)
   contact information 184
   publication
      speech therapy referral 126n
U.S. Food and Drug Administration (FDA)
   contact information 184
   publications
      benefits and risks of cochlear implants 119n
      cochlear implants 118n

U.S. Social Security
    Administration (SSA)
        contact information 184
        publications
            benefits for children with
                disabilities 176n
            qualify for disability
                benefits 178n
USA.gov
    publication
        SSDI and SSI benefits for people
            with disabilities 172n

V

verbal apraxia *see* apraxia of speech
vocal cord paralysis *see* vocal fold
    paralysis
vocal fold hemorrhage, described 26

vocal fold paralysis
    defined 26
    overview 30–32
vocal nodules
    defined 26
    voice problem 21
vocalization *see* voice
voice, defined 3
voice disorders
    described 13
    spasmodic dysphonia 29
    statistics 16
    vocal fold paralysis 26, 30
voice health, overview 20–23
voice therapy
    spasmodic dysphonia 30
    vocal fold paralysis 31
    vocal nodules, polyps, and cysts 26